# BLOOD TYPE A FOOD LIST

A Comprehensive Guide to Enhancing Metabolism with a Diet that Includes Foods to Eat and Avoid

**Patricia D. Stotler**

# Table of Contents

# Introduction

Are You Struggling with Low Energy, Digestive Issues, or Weight Management? Discover How "BLOOD TYPE A FOOD LIST" Can Transform Your Health!

Are you tired of feeling sluggish and bloated after meals? Do you wish you had a clear, personalized guide to help you navigate the confusing world of nutrition? If you have Blood Type A, you might be eating foods that don't suit your unique digestive system. Our book, "BLOOD TYPE A FOOD LIST," is designed to help you unlock the secrets to optimal health tailored specifically to your blood type.

**Benefits of Following the "BLOOD TYPE A FOOD LIST"**

- **Increased Energy Levels:** Feel more energized and productive throughout the day by eating foods that align with your body's needs.
- **Improved Digestion:** Reduce bloating, gas, and other digestive issues by avoiding foods that disrupt your gut.
- **Effective Weight Management:** Achieve and maintain a healthy weight by following a diet plan that works with your metabolism.

- **Enhanced Immunity:** Boost your immune system by eating nutrientrich foods that support your overall health.
- **Better Mental Clarity:** Experience improved focus and concentration by eliminating foods that cause brain fog.

**Overcoming Objections: Why "BLOOD TYPE A FOOD LIST" is the Solution You Need**

**"I've tried other diets before, and they didn't work for me."**

Unlike generic diets, the "BLOOD TYPE A FOOD LIST" is specifically tailored to the unique needs of individuals with Blood Type A. By focusing on foods that are compatible with your genetic makeup, this guide ensures you get the most out of your diet.

**"I don't have time to follow a complicated diet plan."**

Our book provides simple, easytofollow guidelines and meal plans that fit into even the busiest lifestyles. With clear instructions and practical tips, you'll find it easy to incorporate these changes into your daily routine.

**"I'm concerned about missing out on essential nutrients."**

The "BLOOD TYPE A FOOD LIST" emphasizes a balanced diet rich in essential nutrients. We provide detailed information on how to get all the vitamins and minerals you need while avoiding foods that may cause adverse reactions.

**"I don't know how to cook special meals."**

No need to worry! Our book includes a variety of delicious, easytomake recipes that will appeal to your taste buds and suit your nutritional needs. Whether you're a seasoned cook or a kitchen novice, you'll find plenty of meal ideas to enjoy.

**Discover the Story of "BLOOD TYPE A FOOD LIST"**

In a small, bustling town, there was a woman named Emily who struggled with constant fatigue and digestive problems. She tried various diets, hoping to find relief, but nothing seemed to work. Frustrated and at her wit's end, Emily stumbled upon a unique dietary concept: the Blood Type Diet.

Intrigued, she delved into research and discovered the book "BLOOD TYPE A FOOD LIST." This comprehensive guide promised to provide personalized dietary recommendations based on her blood type. Skeptical yet hopeful, Emily decided to give it a try.

As she began to follow the guidelines outlined in the book, Emily noticed remarkable changes. Her energy levels soared, and she no longer felt bloated or uncomfortable after meals. The tailored meal plans were easy to follow, and the recipes were both delicious and nutritious.

Emily's success inspired her to share her story with friends and family, many of whom were also struggling with similar health issues. They, too, experienced the transformative benefits of the "BLOOD TYPE A FOOD LIST." Soon, a community of healthconscious individuals emerged, all thriving on a diet that was perfectly suited to their unique needs.

**Join Emily and countless others on a journey to better health with the "BLOOD TYPE A FOOD LIST." Discover the power of personalized nutrition and unlock your body's full potential.**

# Understanding the Blood Type Diet

## The Science Behind Blood Type Diets

The Blood Type Diet is based on the idea that our blood type affects how our bodies react to certain foods. For individuals with Blood Type A, the diet emphasizes the importance of consuming foods that align with their specific biological and genetic makeup. This diet was popularized by Dr. Peter J. D'Adamo, a naturopathic physician who proposed that different blood types have unique dietary needs.

Individuals with Blood Type A are believed to have evolved from agrarian ancestors who thrived on plant-based diets. As a result, their digestive systems are thought to be more suited to vegetarian or semi-vegetarian diets. This theory suggests that Blood Type A individuals produce lower levels of stomach acid, making it difficult to digest animal proteins and fats efficiently. Consequently, a diet rich in plant-based foods is considered beneficial for their overall health and well-being.

The Blood Type A diet recommends a high intake of vegetables, fruits, legumes, and whole grains. These foods are easier to digest and help maintain an optimal internal environment. Leafy greens, broccoli, carrots, and onions are particularly beneficial as they provide essential vitamins and minerals. Fruits like berries, plums, and cherries are favored due to their antioxidant properties and lower sugar content, which support the immune system and help prevent inflammation.

Legumes such as lentils, black beans, and soy products are excellent sources of protein for Blood Type A individuals. These foods are easier to digest than animal proteins and provide essential nutrients without the associated digestive discomfort. Whole grains like quinoa, brown rice, and oats offer sustained energy and are less likely to cause blood sugar spikes compared to refined grains.

Nuts and seeds, including almonds, walnuts, and flaxseeds, are also recommended for Blood Type A individuals. These provide healthy fats and protein, which support cardiovascular health and help maintain steady energy levels. Olive oil is preferred over other oils due to its anti-inflammatory properties and monounsaturated fat content, which supports heart health.

While the Blood Type A diet emphasizes plant-based foods, it also acknowledges the need for certain animal proteins, albeit in moderation. Poultry, such as chicken and turkey, is considered acceptable in limited quantities. These sources of protein are easier to digest compared to red meat and are less likely to cause adverse reactions. Fish, particularly those rich in omega-3 fatty acids like salmon and sardines, are also recommended due to their anti-inflammatory benefits and positive impact on cardiovascular health.

Dairy products are generally discouraged for Blood Type A individuals. This is due to the lower levels of stomach acid, which make it difficult to digest dairy efficiently. Instead, alternatives such as almond milk, rice milk, and soy milk are suggested. These options provide essential nutrients without causing digestive discomfort.

Wheat and other gluten-containing grains can be problematic for Blood Type A individuals. These grains may contribute to digestive issues and inflammation. As a result, gluten-free grains like quinoa, amaranth, and buckwheat are recommended as suitable alternatives.

The Blood Type A diet also advises avoiding certain foods that can cause negative reactions. These include red meats, processed foods, and certain beans like kidney beans and lima beans, which may inhibit proper nutrient absorption. Additionally, it is suggested to limit the intake of refined sugars and processed foods to maintain stable blood sugar levels and reduce inflammation.

Adopting a diet tailored to Blood Type A can lead to numerous health benefits, including improved digestion, increased energy levels, and enhanced immune function. By focusing on plant-based foods and limiting the intake of foods that are difficult to digest, individuals with Blood Type A can optimize their health and well-being.

Understanding the science behind the Blood Type Diet allows individuals to make informed dietary choices that support their unique biological needs. For those with Blood Type A, this means embracing a diet rich in plant-based foods, moderate amounts of easily digestible animal proteins, and avoiding foods that may cause adverse reactions.

# How Blood Type A Affects Digestion and Metabolism

Blood Type A individuals have a unique set of digestive and metabolic characteristics that influence their overall health and wellness. One of the key aspects of Blood Type A is their relatively low levels of stomach acid. This means that they often struggle to digest animal proteins and fats efficiently. As a result, a diet rich in plant-based proteins, such as tofu and legumes, is typically more beneficial for them. These sources of protein are easier to digest and provide essential nutrients without taxing the digestive system.

Additionally, people with Blood Type A often have a more sensitive immune system. This sensitivity makes them more susceptible to certain illnesses and infections, particularly those related to the respiratory system. To support their immune health, it is crucial for individuals with Blood Type A to consume foods that are rich in antioxidants and other immune-boosting nutrients. Foods such as berries, leafy greens, and garlic are excellent choices for bolstering their immune defenses.

Another important consideration for Blood Type A individuals is their metabolic rate. They tend to have a slower metabolism compared to other blood types. This slower metabolism means that they need to be more mindful of their carbohydrate intake. While whole grains and complex carbohydrates can be beneficial, it is important to avoid refined sugars and processed foods that can lead to weight gain and other metabolic issues. Incorporating a variety of fresh fruits and vegetables can help maintain a balanced metabolism and prevent excess weight gain.

Blood Type A individuals also benefit from regular, moderate exercise. Activities such as yoga, tai chi, and brisk walking are particularly effective in maintaining their physical health and reducing stress levels. High-intensity workouts may not be as suitable for them due to their more delicate cardiovascular and nervous systems. Regular, gentle exercise helps to keep their metabolism active and supports overall well-being.

Fermented foods play a vital role in the diet of Blood Type A individuals. Foods such as yogurt, kefir, and miso provide beneficial probiotics that support gut health. These probiotics are essential for maintaining a healthy balance of gut bacteria, which in turn aids in digestion and nutrient absorption. Given their tendency toward digestive sensitivity, incorporating fermented foods can significantly enhance their digestive efficiency and overall health.

It is also important for Blood Type A individuals to avoid certain foods that can cause adverse reactions. Red meat, dairy products, and certain grains like wheat and corn can be difficult for them to digest and may lead to inflammation and other health issues. Instead, opting for plant-based alternatives, such as almond milk and gluten-free grains like quinoa and amaranth, can help mitigate these issues and promote better digestive health.

Blood Type A individuals should also be cautious with their intake of stimulants such as caffeine and alcohol. These substances can exacerbate stress and anxiety, which are already common concerns for people with this blood type. Herbal teas and plenty of water are better choices for staying hydrated and maintaining a calm, balanced state of mind.

By understanding the specific needs of Blood Type A individuals, it becomes clear why a tailored diet is so important. The Blood Type A Food List provides a comprehensive guide to selecting foods that support their unique digestive and metabolic requirements. This approach not only enhances physical health but also promotes a sense of overall well-being and vitality.

# Benefits of Following a Blood Type A Diet

Following a Blood Type A diet offers numerous benefits that cater specifically to the unique needs of individuals with Blood Type A. By adhering to a diet that aligns with your genetic makeup, you can experience improved overall health and well-being.

One of the primary benefits is increased energy levels. Individuals with Blood Type A often struggle with low energy and fatigue due to their body's unique metabolic processes. By consuming foods that are compatible with their blood type, they can optimize their energy production and feel more vibrant and active throughout the day.

Improved digestion is another significant advantage. Blood Type A individuals tend to have a more sensitive digestive system. By avoiding foods that cause irritation or discomfort, such as certain meats and dairy products, they can reduce symptoms like bloating, gas, and indigestion. Instead, incorporating easily digestible foods like vegetables, fruits, and plant-based proteins helps maintain a healthy digestive tract.

Effective weight management becomes more achievable when following a Blood Type A diet. This diet emphasizes foods that support a balanced metabolism, making it easier to achieve and maintain a healthy weight. By focusing on lean proteins, whole grains, and fresh produce, individuals can create a sustainable eating pattern that prevents weight gain and promotes fat loss.

Enhanced immunity is another benefit, as the diet includes foods rich in vitamins, minerals, and antioxidants that support the immune system. Blood Type A individuals are more prone to infections and illnesses, so consuming nutrient-dense foods like leafy greens, berries, and nuts can help boost their immune defenses and improve their overall health.

Better mental clarity and focus are also notable benefits. Certain foods that are incompatible with Blood Type A can cause brain fog and hinder cognitive function. By eliminating these foods and consuming those that promote brain health, such as omega-3 rich fish, nuts, and seeds, individuals can experience improved concentration and mental sharpness.

The Blood Type A diet also promotes cardiovascular health. By focusing on plant-based proteins and healthy fats, it helps reduce cholesterol levels and lower the risk of heart disease. Foods like soy, olive oil, and avocados provide essential nutrients that support heart health and improve circulation.

Stress reduction is another advantage, as the diet encourages the consumption of calming foods that help regulate stress hormones. Incorporating foods like tofu, green vegetables, and herbal teas can aid in managing stress and promoting a sense of calm and well-being.

By following the Blood Type A diet outlined in the BLOOD TYPE A FOOD LIST, individuals can experience these comprehensive benefits, leading to a healthier, more balanced lifestyle tailored to their unique genetic needs.

# Overview of the Blood Type A Diet

## Historical Background and Evolutionary Theory

The Blood Type A diet is grounded in the idea that different blood types have evolved to thrive on specific types of diets, reflecting the dietary habits and environments of our ancestors. The historical background and evolutionary theory behind the Blood Type A diet provide a fascinating insight into how our genetic makeup influences our nutritional needs.

According to this theory, Blood Type A is associated with the advent of agriculture, which began around 10,000 years ago. This period marked a significant shift in human history, as societies transitioned from hunter-gatherer lifestyles to settled farming communities. As a result, people with Blood Type A are believed to have adapted to a diet that is more plant-based, reflecting the agricultural products that became staples in these early farming societies.

The evolutionary perspective suggests that Blood Type A individuals have a digestive system that is optimized for processing grains, vegetables, and fruits. This adaptation is thought to result from the need to efficiently metabolize the carbohydrate-rich foods that were prevalent in agricultural societies. The diet recommends a variety of plant-based foods that are easily digestible and provide essential nutrients without causing inflammation or other digestive issues.

Moreover, the theory posits that Blood Type A individuals have a naturally lower level of stomach acid compared to other blood types. This means that they may struggle to digest animal proteins and fats efficiently, which can lead to digestive discomfort and other health issues. Therefore, the diet emphasizes plant-based proteins, such as tofu, beans, and legumes, which are easier for Blood Type A individuals to digest and assimilate.

The historical context also explains why Blood Type A individuals might benefit from avoiding certain foods. For example, red meat is considered difficult for them to digest, potentially leading to an increased risk of heart disease and cancer. Dairy products are also recommended to be limited, as they can cause digestive problems due to the lower levels of stomach acid. Instead, the diet encourages the consumption of fermented dairy products like yogurt and kefir, which are easier to digest and provide beneficial probiotics.

The evolutionary theory further extends to lifestyle factors. Blood Type A individuals are thought to thrive on a balanced lifestyle that includes regular, moderate exercise and stress management practices. This reflects the stable and community-oriented life of early agricultural societies, where physical labor was constant but not excessively strenuous, and social cohesion was essential for survival.

In essence, the Blood Type A diet is built on the premise that our evolutionary history has shaped our genetic predispositions, including our optimal dietary patterns. By aligning our modern eating habits with the diet that our ancestors adapted to, individuals with Blood Type A can potentially enhance their overall health and well-being. This approach not only honors the wisdom of our evolutionary past but also provides a practical framework for achieving a balanced and nutritious diet in the present day.

# Key Principles of the Blood Type A Diet

The Blood Type A Diet is based on the idea that individuals with different blood types process foods differently and that these differences can impact their overall health and well-being. For those with Blood Type A, the diet emphasizes consuming foods that are naturally suited to their body's needs, promoting optimal digestion, enhanced energy levels, and improved immune function.

One of the core principles of the Blood Type A Diet is the focus on plant-based foods. People with Blood Type A generally thrive on a diet rich in vegetables, fruits, legumes, and whole grains. This aligns with the belief that Blood Type A individuals have a digestive system that is better suited to a vegetarian or near-vegetarian lifestyle. The inclusion of organic, fresh produce is highly recommended to minimize the intake of pesticides and other chemicals that could potentially disrupt the digestive system.

Protein sources in the Blood Type A Diet should primarily come from plant-based options, such as tofu, tempeh, and other soy products, as well as beans and legumes. While fish and seafood are also acceptable, it is advised to avoid most meats, particularly red meats, as they can be harder to digest and may contribute to various health issues. Poultry can be consumed in moderation, but it should not be a primary protein source.

Another key principle is the avoidance of dairy products. Blood Type A individuals often have difficulty digesting lactose, which can lead to digestive discomfort and other related issues. Instead of dairy, the diet encourages the consumption of alternatives such as almond milk, soy milk, and other plant-based dairy substitutes. These alternatives provide similar nutritional benefits without the adverse effects associated with traditional dairy products.

Grains and cereals play an essential role in the Blood Type A Diet. Whole grains such as quinoa, amaranth, and spelt are preferred over processed grains and wheat products, which can cause inflammation and digestive problems. Incorporating a variety of whole grains ensures a well-rounded intake of fiber, vitamins, and minerals, supporting overall digestive health and providing sustained energy.

Healthy fats are also an important component of the Blood Type A Diet. Olive oil, flaxseed oil, and other plant-based oils are recommended for their beneficial effects on heart health and overall well-being. These oils can be used in cooking, dressings, and marinades, providing a flavorful and nutritious addition to meals.

The diet also emphasizes the importance of avoiding certain foods that can be detrimental to those with Blood Type A. These include processed foods, refined sugars, and artificial additives, which can lead to inflammation, weight gain, and other health problems. Additionally, specific vegetables like tomatoes, peppers, and eggplants are advised against due to their potential to cause digestive issues and inflammation.

Stress management and regular physical activity are integral to the Blood Type A lifestyle. It is believed that individuals with Blood Type A tend to be more sensitive to stress, which can negatively impact their health. Incorporating stress-reducing activities such as yoga, meditation, and tai chi can help maintain balance and promote overall wellness. Regular, moderate exercise like walking, swimming, and cycling is also recommended to support cardiovascular health and maintain a healthy weight.

The Blood Type A Diet encourages mindfulness in eating habits, promoting the idea of listening to one's body and eating in a relaxed, peaceful environment. This approach helps individuals tune into their hunger cues, avoid overeating, and enjoy their meals more thoroughly.

By adhering to the principles of the Blood Type A Diet, individuals can experience a range of health benefits, including improved digestion, increased energy levels, and a strengthened immune system. The diet provides a holistic approach to nutrition that is tailored to the specific needs of those with Blood Type A, fostering long-term health and well-being.

# Essential Nutritional Needs

## Macronutrient Breakdown

For individuals with Blood Type A, macronutrient balance is crucial for optimizing health and wellness. The diet emphasizes plant-based foods, which align with the genetic predisposition of Blood Type A individuals towards a more agrarian lifestyle. The primary macronutrients to focus on are proteins, carbohydrates, and fats, each playing a distinct role in maintaining overall health.

Proteins for Blood Type A should come predominantly from plant-based sources. This includes beans, legumes, tofu, and tempeh. These sources are easier to digest and provide ample protein without the inflammatory effects that some animal proteins can have on individuals with Blood Type A. Occasionally, fish and seafood can be included, as they offer beneficial omega-3 fatty acids and are typically easier to digest than red meat or poultry. However, red meat and poultry are generally recommended to be minimized or avoided due to potential digestive difficulties and adverse health effects.

Carbohydrates should primarily come from vegetables, fruits, and whole grains. Vegetables are particularly beneficial, offering a wide range of vitamins, minerals, and fiber while being low in calories. Leafy greens, carrots, broccoli, and other non-starchy vegetables are highly recommended. Fruits such as berries, apples, and plums provide essential vitamins and antioxidants. Whole grains like quinoa, brown rice, and oats are preferred over refined grains, as they maintain their nutritional integrity and offer more fiber, aiding in digestion and maintaining stable blood sugar levels.

Fats are an essential part of the diet but should be sourced carefully. Healthy fats from olive oil, flaxseed oil, and certain nuts like walnuts and almonds are beneficial. These fats provide essential fatty acids that support cardiovascular health and help in the absorption of fat-soluble vitamins. It is advisable to avoid or limit saturated fats and trans fats found in processed foods, as they can contribute to inflammation and other health issues.

In summary, the macronutrient breakdown for Blood Type A emphasizes a diet rich in plant-based proteins, complex carbohydrates from vegetables, fruits, and whole grains, and healthy fats from natural sources. This approach helps to align dietary practices with the unique digestive and metabolic needs of individuals with Blood Type A, promoting better overall health and wellness.

# Micronutrient Essentials

For individuals with Blood Type A, focusing on micronutrient essentials is crucial to optimize health and well-being. These essential nutrients play a vital role in various bodily functions, including immune support, energy production, and cellular repair. To ensure you receive adequate micronutrients, it is important to incorporate specific foods into your diet that align with the Blood Type A dietary recommendations.

Vitamin A is a key micronutrient for Blood Type A individuals. It supports immune function, vision, and skin health. Foods rich in beta-carotene, a precursor to vitamin A, are particularly beneficial. These include carrots, sweet potatoes, and leafy green vegetables like spinach and kale. Including these vegetables in your diet can help maintain optimal vitamin A levels.

Vitamin C is another essential nutrient, known for its immune-boosting properties and role in collagen synthesis. Blood Type A individuals should focus on consuming fruits and vegetables that are high in vitamin C but gentle on the digestive system. Berries, such as strawberries and blueberries, as well as citrus fruits like oranges and grapefruits, are excellent sources. Bell peppers and broccoli also provide a significant amount of vitamin C and are suitable for Blood Type A.

Folate, a B vitamin, is crucial for DNA synthesis and repair, making it essential for overall cellular health. Leafy green vegetables, such as spinach and romaine lettuce, are rich in folate and highly recommended for Blood Type A. Legumes like lentils and chickpeas are also excellent sources of folate and fit well within the dietary guidelines.

Iron is vital for oxygen transport and energy production. While Blood Type A individuals may need to avoid red meat, which is a common source of iron, they can obtain this nutrient from plant-based sources. Spinach, lentils, and tofu are all rich in non-heme iron, which can be effectively absorbed when paired with vitamin C-rich foods. This combination enhances iron absorption and supports overall energy levels.

Calcium is necessary for bone health and nerve function. Blood Type A individuals should seek out plant-based sources of calcium, as dairy products are not typically recommended. Leafy greens like kale, collard greens, and broccoli are excellent choices. Additionally, fortified plant-based milk alternatives, such as almond milk and soy milk, can provide a significant amount of calcium.

Magnesium plays a critical role in muscle and nerve function, blood sugar control, and bone health. Nuts and seeds, such as almonds, sunflower seeds, and flaxseeds, are rich in magnesium and align well with the Blood Type A diet. Whole grains, including quinoa and oats, also provide substantial amounts of magnesium and should be included in your daily meals.

Zinc is essential for immune function, wound healing, and protein synthesis. Blood Type A individuals can obtain zinc from plant-based sources like pumpkin seeds, sesame seeds, and chickpeas. Including these foods in your diet ensures adequate zinc intake without the need for animal products that may not align with Blood Type A dietary recommendations.

Omega-3 fatty acids are important for heart health, reducing inflammation, and supporting brain function. Blood Type A individuals are encouraged to consume fish, such as salmon and mackerel, which are rich in omega-3s. For those following a vegetarian or vegan diet, chia seeds, flaxseeds, and walnuts are excellent plant-based sources of omega-3 fatty acids.

By focusing on these micronutrient essentials and incorporating the recommended foods into your diet, Blood Type A individuals can achieve a balanced and nutritious dietary plan. Ensuring adequate intake of these vitamins and minerals supports overall health, enhances energy levels, and promotes optimal bodily functions.

# Food Groups to Eat

## Vegetables

| Vegetable | Nutritional Information (per 100g serving) | Serving Size | Cooking Instructions | Cooking Time |
| --- | --- | --- | --- | --- |
| Broccoli | 34 calories, 2.8g protein, 6.4g carbs | 1 cup chopped | Steam until tender | 5-7 minutes |
| Spinach | 23 calories, 2.9g protein, 3.6g carbs | 1 cup leaves | Sauté with olive oil | 2-3 minutes |
| Kale | 49 calories, 4.3g protein, 8.8g carbs | 1 cup chopped | Bake into chips | 10-15 minutes |
| Carrots | 41 calories, 0.9g protein, 9.6g carbs | 1 medium carrot | Boil or roast | 10-15 minutes |
| Sweet Potatoes | 86 calories, 1.6g protein, | 1 small potato | Bake or microwave | 45 minutes (bake), 5-7 |

| Vegetable | Nutritional Information (per 100g serving) | Serving Size | Cooking Instructions | Cooking Time |
|---|---|---|---|---|
|  | 20g carbs |  |  | minutes (microwave) |
| Garlic | 149 calories, 6.4g protein, 33g carbs | 1 clove | Add minced to dishes | Cook with dish |
| Onions | 40 calories, 1.1g protein, 9.3g carbs | 1 medium onion | Sauté until caramelized | 10-15 minutes |
| Red Bell Peppers | 31 calories, 1g protein, 6g carbs | 1 medium pepper | Grill or roast | 10-15 minutes |
| Pumpkin | 26 calories, 1g protein, 6.5g carbs | 1 cup cubes | Roast or make into soup | 30 minutes (roast) |
| Beets | 43 calories, 1.6g protein, 10g carbs | 1 medium beet | Boil or roast | 30-40 minutes |
| Artichokes | 47 calories, 3.3g protein, | 1 medium | Steam or boil | 25-45 minutes |

| Vegetable | Nutritional Information (per 100g serving) | Serving Size | Cooking Instructions | Cooking Time |
| --- | --- | --- | --- | --- |
| | 11g carbs | artichoke | | |
| Collard Greens | 32 calories, 3g protein, 5.4g carbs | 1 cup chopped | Sauté with garlic | 5-7 minutes |
| Swiss Chard | 19 calories, 1.8g protein, 3.7g carbs | 1 cup chopped | Sauté lightly | 3-5 minutes |
| Parsley | 36 calories, 3g protein, 6.3g carbs | 1 cup chopped | Use fresh as garnish | No cook |
| Zucchini | 17 calories, 1.2g protein, 3.1g carbs | 1 medium zucchini | Grill or sauté | 5-10 minutes |

Each vegetable listed is particularly beneficial for Blood Type A due to its compatibility with the digestive system and immune response characteristics of this blood type. These vegetables can be incorporated into meals in various ways to ensure a balanced intake of nutrients, enhancing overall health and well-being for individuals with Blood Type A. The serving sizes and cooking times provided allow for optimal preservation of nutrients and flavors, making these vegetables both a healthy and tasty addition to your diet.

# Fruits

| Fruit | Ingredients | Instructions | Nutritional Information | Serving Size | Cooking Time |
|---|---|---|---|---|---|
| Blueberries | 1 cup fresh blueberries | Rinse under cold water and enjoy fresh. | Calories: 85, Carbs: 21g, Fiber: 4g, Vitamin C: 24% DV, Vitamin K: 36% DV, Antioxidants: High | 1 cup | 0 minutes |
| Strawberries | 1 cup fresh strawberries | Rinse, hull, and slice if desired. Enjoy fresh or add to salads. | Calories: 49, Carbs: 12g, Fiber: 3g, Vitamin C: 149% DV, Folate: 9% DV, Antioxidants: High | 1 cup | 0 minutes |

| Fruit | Ingredients | Instructions | Nutritional Information | Serving Size | Cooking Time |
| --- | --- | --- | --- | --- | --- |
| Oranges | 1 medium orange | Peel and separate into segments. Enjoy fresh or add to salads. | Calories: 62, Carbs: 15g, Fiber: 3g, Vitamin C: 116% DV, Folate: 10% DV | 1 medium | 0 minutes |
| Grapefruits | 1 medium grapefruit | Peel and segment. Enjoy fresh or add to salads. | Calories: 52, Carbs: 13g, Fiber: 2g, Vitamin C: 64% DV, Vitamin A: 28% DV | 1 medium | 0 minutes |
| Cherries | 1 cup fresh cherries | Rinse and pit if needed. Enjoy fresh or add to desserts. | Calories: 97, Carbs: 25g, Fiber: 3g, Vitamin C: 18% DV, Potassium: 10% DV | 1 cup | 0 minutes |

| Fruit | Ingredients | Instructions | Nutritional Information | Serving Size | Cooking Time |
| --- | --- | --- | --- | --- | --- |
| Kiwi | 2 medium kiwis | Peel and slice. Enjoy fresh or add to fruit salads. | Calories: 84, Carbs: 20g, Fiber: 4g, Vitamin C: 278% DV, Vitamin K: 46% DV, Potassium: 14% DV | 2 medium | 0 minutes |
| Pineapple | 1 cup fresh pineapple | Peel, core, and cut into chunks. Enjoy fresh or add to salads. | Calories: 82, Carbs: 22g, Fiber: 2g, Vitamin C: 131% DV, Manganese: 76% DV | 1 cup | 0 minutes |
| Mango | 1 medium mango | Peel and cut into slices or chunks. Enjoy fresh or add to | Calories: 202, Carbs: 50g, Fiber: 5g, Vitamin C: 203% | 1 medium | 0 minutes |

| Fruit | Ingredients | Instructions | Nutritional Information | Serving Size | Cooking Time |
|---|---|---|---|---|---|
|  |  | salads. | DV, Vitamin A: 72% DV, Folate: 20% DV |  |  |
| Papaya | 1 cup fresh papaya | Peel, remove seeds, and cut into chunks. Enjoy fresh or add to salads. | Calories: 55, Carbs: 14g, Fiber: 3g, Vitamin C: 144% DV, Vitamin A: 31% DV, Folate: 13% DV | 1 cup | 0 minutes |
| Peaches | 1 medium peach | Rinse, pit, and slice. Enjoy fresh or add to salads. | Calories: 59, Carbs: 15g, Fiber: 2g, Vitamin C: 17% DV, Vitamin A: 10% DV | 1 medium | 0 minutes |

| Fruit | Ingredients | Instructions | Nutritional Information | Serving Size | Cooking Time |
|---|---|---|---|---|---|
| Plums | 2 medium plums | Rinse, pit, and slice. Enjoy fresh or add to salads. | Calories: 60, Carbs: 16g, Fiber: 2g, Vitamin C: 15% DV, Vitamin K: 10% DV, Antioxidants: High | 2 medium | 0 minutes |
| Apricots | 4 fresh apricots | Rinse, pit, and slice. Enjoy fresh or add to salads. | Calories: 34, Carbs: 8g, Fiber: 1g, Vitamin A: 13% DV, Vitamin C: 8% DV | 4 apricots | 0 minutes |
| Apples | 1 medium apple | Rinse and slice. Enjoy fresh or add to salads. | Calories: 95, Carbs: 25g, Fiber: 4g, Vitamin C: 14% DV, | 1 medium | 0 minutes |

| Fruit | Ingredients | Instructions | Nutritional Information | Serving Size | Cooking Time |
|---|---|---|---|---|---|
| | | | Potassium: 6% DV | | |
| Pears | 1 medium pear | Rinse and slice. Enjoy fresh or add to salads. | Calories: 101, Carbs: 27g, Fiber: 6g, Vitamin C: 12% DV, Vitamin K: 10% DV | 1 medium | 0 minutes |
| Grapes | 1 cup fresh grapes | Rinse and enjoy fresh. Add to salads or cheese plates. | Calories: 62, Carbs: 16g, Fiber: 1g, Vitamin C: 6% DV, Vitamin K: 18% DV | 1 cup | 0 minutes |

These fruits are not only delicious but also packed with essential nutrients that support the health and well-being of individuals with Blood Type A. Incorporating a variety of these fruits into your daily diet ensures you receive a wide range of vitamins, minerals, and antioxidants, which contribute to overall health and vitality. Enjoy these fruits fresh for the best nutritional benefits and flavor.

# Grains and Cereals

| Grain/Cereal | Ingredients | Instructions | Nutritional Information | Serving Size | Cooking Time |
|---|---|---|---|---|---|
| Quinoa | 1 cup quinoa, 2 cups water | Rinse quinoa. Boil water, add quinoa, reduce heat, cover, simmer for 15 minutes. Fluff with fork. | Calories: 222, Protein: 8g, Fiber: 5g | 1 cup cooked | 15 minutes |
| Brown Rice | 1 cup brown rice, 2 ½ cups water | Rinse rice. Boil water, add rice, reduce heat, cover, simmer for 45 minutes. | Calories: 216, Protein: 5g, Fiber: 3.5g | 1 cup cooked | 45 minutes |

| Grain/Cereal | Ingredients | Instructions | Nutritional Information | Serving Size | Cooking Time |
|---|---|---|---|---|---|
| | | Let stand 10 minutes, fluff with fork. | | | |
| Oats | 1 cup rolled oats, 2 cups water or milk | Boil water or milk, add oats, reduce heat, simmer for 10 minutes, stirring occasionally. | Calories: 154, Protein: 6g, Fiber: 4g | 1 cup cooked | 10 minutes |
| Millet | 1 cup millet, 2 cups water | Toast millet in dry pan, add water, bring to boil, reduce heat, cover, simmer for | Calories: 207, Protein: 6g, Fiber: 2.3g | 1 cup cooked | 20 minutes |

| Grain/Cereal | Ingredients | Instructions | Nutritional Information | Serving Size | Cooking Time |
|---|---|---|---|---|---|
| | | 20 minutes. Fluff with fork. | | | |
| Amaranth | 1 cup amaranth, 2 ½ cups water | Boil water, add amaranth, reduce heat, cover, simmer for 20 minutes, stirring occasionally. | Calories: 251, Protein: 9g, Fiber: 5g | 1 cup cooked | 20 minutes |
| Spelt | 1 cup spelt, 3 cups water | Soak spelt overnight, drain. Boil water, add spelt, reduce heat, | Calories: 246, Protein: 11g, Fiber: 7.6g | 1 cup cooked | 50 minutes |

| Grain/Cereal | Ingredients | Instructions | Nutritional Information | Serving Size | Cooking Time |
|---|---|---|---|---|---|
|  |  | simmer for 50 minutes, drain excess water. |  |  |  |
| Barley | 1 cup pearl barley, 3 cups water | Rinse barley. Boil water, add barley, reduce heat, simmer for 45 minutes, drain excess water. | Calories: 193, Protein: 3.5g, Fiber: 6g | 1 cup cooked | 45 minutes |
| Teff | 1 cup teff, 3 cups water | Boil water, add teff, reduce heat, cover, simmer for 20 minutes, stirring | Calories: 255, Protein: 9.75g, Fiber: 7g | 1 cup cooked | 20 minutes |

| Grain/Cereal | Ingredients | Instructions | Nutritional Information | Serving Size | Cooking Time |
| --- | --- | --- | --- | --- | --- |
| | | occasionally. | | | |
| Rye | 1 cup rye berries, 3 cups water | Soak rye berries overnight, drain. Boil water, add rye, reduce heat, simmer for 1 hour, drain excess water. | Calories: 340, Protein: 10g, Fiber: 24g | 1 cup cooked | 1 hour |
| Buckwheat | 1 cup buckwheat groats, 2 cups water | Rinse buckwheat. Boil water, add buckwheat, reduce heat, simmer for | Calories: 155, Protein: 5.7g, Fiber: 4.5g | 1 cup cooked | 20 minutes |

| Grain/Cereal | Ingredients | Instructions | Nutritional Information | Serving Size | Cooking Time |
|---|---|---|---|---|---|
| | | 20 minutes. Fluff with fork. | | | |
| Farro | 1 cup farro, 3 cups water | Rinse farro. Boil water, add farro, reduce heat, simmer for 30 minutes, drain excess water. | Calories: 200, Protein: 7g, Fiber: 3g | 1 cup cooked | 30 minutes |
| Kamut | 1 cup kamut, 4 cups water | Soak kamut overnight, drain. Boil water, add kamut, reduce heat, simmer for 40 minutes, drain excess | Calories: 251, Protein: 11g, Fiber: 7.4g | 1 cup cooked | 40 minutes |

| Grain/Cereal | Ingredients | Instructions | Nutritional Information | Serving Size | Cooking Time |
|---|---|---|---|---|---|
| | | water. | | | |
| Sorghum | 1 cup sorghum, 3 cups water | Rinse sorghum. Boil water, add sorghum, reduce heat, cover, simmer for 50-60 minutes, drain excess water. | Calories: 329, Protein: 10.6g, Fiber: 12g | 1 cup cooked | 50-60 minutes |
| Freekeh | 1 cup freekeh, 2 ½ cups water | Rinse freekeh. Boil water, add freekeh, reduce heat, cover, | Calories: 200, Protein: 8g, Fiber: 4g | 1 cup cooked | 20 minutes |

| Grain/Cereal | Ingredients | Instructions | Nutritional Information | Serving Size | Cooking Time |
|---|---|---|---|---|---|
| | | simmer for 20 minutes, drain excess water. | | | |
| Wild Rice | 1 cup wild rice, 4 cups water | Rinse wild rice. Boil water, add rice, reduce heat, cover, simmer for 45 minutes, drain excess water. | Calories: 166, Protein: 6.5g, Fiber: 3g | 1 cup cooked | 45 minutes |

# Legumes and Beans

| Legume/Bean | Ingredient | Instructions | Nutritional Information (Per Serving) | Serving Size | Cooking Time |
| --- | --- | --- | --- | --- | --- |
| Black Beans | 1 cup dried black beans | Rinse beans. Soak overnight. Cook in fresh water for 60-90 minutes until tender. | Calories: 227, Protein: 15g, Fiber: 15g, Iron: 3.6mg | 1 cup cooked | Soak: Overnight, Cook: 60-90 min |
| Lentils | 1 cup dried green lentils | Rinse lentils. Cook in 3 cups water for 20-25 minutes until | Calories: 230, Protein: 18g, Fiber: 15.6g, Iron: 6.6mg | 1 cup cooked | 20-25 min |

| Legume/Bean | Ingredient | Instructions | Nutritional Information (Per Serving) | Serving Size | Cooking Time |
|---|---|---|---|---|---|
| | | tender. | | | |
| Chickpeas | 1 cup dried chickpeas | Rinse chickpeas. Soak overnight. Cook in fresh water for 60-90 minutes until tender. | Calories: 269, Protein: 14.5g, Fiber: 12.5g, Iron: 4.7mg | 1 cup cooked | Soak: Overnight, Cook: 60-90 min |
| Black-eyed Peas | 1 cup dried black-eyed peas | Rinse peas. Soak for 2 hours. Cook in fresh water for 45-60 | Calories: 200, Protein: 13g, Fiber: 11g, Iron: 4.3mg | 1 cup cooked | Soak: 2 hours, Cook: 45-60 min |

| Legume/Bean | Ingredient | Instructions | Nutritional Information (Per Serving) | Serving Size | Cooking Time |
|---|---|---|---|---|---|
| | | minutes until tender. | | | |
| Adzuki Beans | 1 cup dried adzuki beans | Rinse beans. Soak for 1-2 hours. Cook in fresh water for 45-60 minutes until tender. | Calories: 294, Protein: 17g, Fiber: 13g, Iron: 4.6mg | 1 cup cooked | Soak: 1-2 hours, Cook: 45-60 min |
| Navy Beans | 1 cup dried navy beans | Rinse beans. Soak overnight. Cook in fresh water for 60-90 | Calories: 255, Protein: 15g, Fiber: 19g, Iron: 4.3mg | 1 cup cooked | Soak: Overnight, Cook: 60-90 min |

| Legume/Bean | Ingredient | Instructions | Nutritional Information (Per Serving) | Serving Size | Cooking Time |
| --- | --- | --- | --- | --- | --- |
| | | minutes until tender. | | | |
| Kidney Beans | 1 cup dried kidney beans | Rinse beans. Soak overnight. Cook in fresh water for 60-90 minutes until tender. | Calories: 225, Protein: 15g, Fiber: 13g, Iron: 3.9mg | 1 cup cooked | Soak: Overnight, Cook: 60-90 min |
| Pinto Beans | 1 cup dried pinto beans | Rinse beans. Soak overnight. Cook in fresh water for 60-90 | Calories: 245, Protein: 15g, Fiber: 15g, Iron: 3.6mg | 1 cup cooked | Soak: Overnight, Cook: 60-90 min |

| Legume/Bean | Ingredient | Instructions | Nutritional Information (Per Serving) | Serving Size | Cooking Time |
| --- | --- | --- | --- | --- | --- |
| | | minutes until tender. | | | |
| Lima Beans | 1 cup dried lima beans | Rinse beans. Soak overnight. Cook in fresh water for 60-90 minutes until tender. | Calories: 209, Protein: 12g, Fiber: 13g, Iron: 4.5mg | 1 cup cooked | Soak: Overnight, Cook: 60-90 min |
| Mung Beans | 1 cup dried mung beans | Rinse beans. Soak for 4 hours. Cook in fresh water for 45-60 | Calories: 212, Protein: 14g, Fiber: 15g, Iron: 3.6mg | 1 cup cooked | Soak: 4 hours, Cook: 45-60 min |

| Legume/Bean | Ingredient | Instructions | Nutritional Information (Per Serving) | Serving Size | Cooking Time |
|---|---|---|---|---|---|
| | | minutes until tender. | | | |
| Cannellini Beans | 1 cup dried cannellini beans | Rinse beans. Soak overnight. Cook in fresh water for 60-90 minutes until tender. | Calories: 225, Protein: 15g, Fiber: 11g, Iron: 4.3mg | 1 cup cooked | Soak: Overnight, Cook: 60-90 min |
| Fava Beans | 1 cup dried fava beans | Rinse beans. Soak overnight. Cook in fresh water for 60-90 | Calories: 187, Protein: 13g, Fiber: 9g, Iron: 2.1mg | 1 cup cooked | Soak: Overnight, Cook: 60-90 min |

| Legume/Bean | Ingredient | Instructions | Nutritional Information (Per Serving) | Serving Size | Cooking Time |
|---|---|---|---|---|---|
|  |  | minutes until tender. |  |  |  |
| Great Northern Beans | 1 cup dried Great Northern beans | Rinse beans. Soak overnight. Cook in fresh water for 60-90 minutes until tender. | Calories: 209, Protein: 14g, Fiber: 12g, Iron: 3.6mg | 1 cup cooked | Soak: Overnight, Cook: 60-90 min |
| Green Peas | 1 cup dried green peas | Rinse peas. Soak for 2 hours. Cook in fresh water for 30-40 | Calories: 231, Protein: 16g, Fiber: 15g, Iron: 2.1mg | 1 cup cooked | Soak: 2 hours, Cook: 30-40 min |

| Legume/Bean | Ingredient | Instructions | Nutritional Information (Per Serving) | Serving Size | Cooking Time |
|---|---|---|---|---|---|
| | | minutes until tender. | | | |
| Red Lentils | 1 cup dried red lentils | Rinse lentils. Cook in 3 cups water for 15-20 minutes until tender. | Calories: 230, Protein: 18g, Fiber: 15.6g, Iron: 6.6mg | 1 cup cooked | 15-20 min |

Each of these legumes and beans is beneficial for Blood Type A individuals due to their high fiber content, protein, and essential nutrients such as iron and folate. Incorporating these into your diet can enhance overall health, improve digestion, and provide a substantial source of plant-based protein.

# Nuts and Seeds

| Nut/Seed | Ingredients | Instructions | Nutritional Information (per serving) | Serving Size | Cooking Time |
|---|---|---|---|---|---|
| Almonds | Raw almonds | Enjoy raw or lightly toasted. Add to salads, oatmeal, or yogurt. | 160 calories, 6g protein, 14g fat, 6g carbs, 3g fiber | 1 ounce (28g) | 5 minutes (toasting) |
| Walnuts | Raw walnuts | Eat raw as a snack or add to baked goods, salads, or oatmeal. | 185 calories, 4g protein, 18g fat, 4g carbs, 2g fiber | 1 ounce (28g) | N/A |

| Nut/Seed | Ingredients | Instructions | Nutritional Information (per serving) | Serving Size | Cooking Time |
| --- | --- | --- | --- | --- | --- |
| Pumpkin Seeds | Raw pumpkin seeds | Eat raw or roast with a pinch of salt. Sprinkle over salads or soups. | 151 calories, 7g protein, 13g fat, 5g carbs, 1g fiber | 1 ounce (28g) | 15 minutes (roasting) |
| Flaxseeds | Whole or ground flaxseeds | Add ground flaxseeds to smoothies, oatmeal, or baked goods. Use whole seeds as a crunchy topping. | 150 calories, 5g protein, 12g fat, 8g carbs, 8g fiber | 2 tablespoons | N/A |

| Nut/Seed | Ingredients | Instructions | Nutritional Information (per serving) | Serving Size | Cooking Time |
|---|---|---|---|---|---|
| Chia Seeds | Raw chia seeds | Mix into smoothies, yogurt, or make chia pudding by soaking in liquid overnight. | 137 calories, 4g protein, 9g fat, 12g carbs, 10g fiber | 1 ounce (28g) | N/A |
| Sunflower Seeds | Raw or roasted sunflower seeds | Eat raw, roasted, or add to salads and baked goods. | 165 calories, 6g protein, 14g fat, 7g carbs, 3g fiber | 1 ounce (28g) | 15 minutes (roasting) |
| Sesame Seeds | Raw sesame seeds | Sprinkle on salads, stir-fries, or baked goods. | 160 calories, 5g protein, 14g fat, 7g carbs, 4g | 2 tablespoons | N/A |

| Nut/Seed | Ingredients | Instructions | Nutritional Information (per serving) | Serving Size | Cooking Time |
|---|---|---|---|---|---|
|  |  |  | fiber |  |  |
| Hemp Seeds | Raw hemp seeds | Add to smoothies, yogurt, or salads. | 166 calories, 10g protein, 14g fat, 2g carbs, 1g fiber | 3 tablespoons | N/A |
| Cashews | Raw or lightly toasted cashews | Enjoy raw, toasted, or in stir-fries and curries. | 155 calories, 5g protein, 12g fat, 9g carbs, 1g fiber | 1 ounce (28g) | 10 minutes (toasting) |
| Pistachios | Raw or lightly salted pistachios | Eat raw, roasted, or add to salads and | 159 calories, 6g protein, 13g fat, 8g | 1 ounce (28g) | N/A |

| Nut/Seed | Ingredients | Instructions | Nutritional Information (per serving) | Serving Size | Cooking Time |
| --- | --- | --- | --- | --- | --- |
| | | desserts. | carbs, 3g fiber | | |
| Pecan Nuts | Raw pecan nuts | Eat raw, toasted, or add to baked goods and salads. | 200 calories, 3g protein, 20g fat, 4g carbs, 3g fiber | 1 ounce (28g) | 10 minutes (toasting) |
| Brazil Nuts | Raw Brazil nuts | Eat raw as a snack or chop and add to salads and desserts. | 187 calories, 4g protein, 19g fat, 3g carbs, 2g fiber | 1 ounce (28g) | N/A |
| Macadamia Nuts | Raw or lightly toasted macadamia | Eat raw, toasted, or add to baked | 204 calories, 2g protein, 21g fat, 4g | 1 ounce (28g) | 10 minutes (toasting) |

| Nut/Seed | Ingredients | Instructions | Nutritional Information (per serving) | Serving Size | Cooking Time |
|---|---|---|---|---|---|
| | nuts | goods and salads. | carbs, 2g fiber | | |
| Pine Nuts | Raw pine nuts | Eat raw, toasted, or add to pesto, salads, and baked goods. | 191 calories, 4g protein, 19g fat, 4g carbs, 1g fiber | 1 ounce (28g) | 5 minutes (toasting) |
| Hazelnuts | Raw or lightly toasted hazelnuts | Eat raw, toasted, or add to baked goods and salads. | 178 calories, 4g protein, 17g fat, 5g carbs, 3g fiber | 1 ounce (28g) | 10 minutes (toasting) |

Incorporating these nuts and seeds into your daily diet can provide essential nutrients, healthy fats, and protein that align with the Blood

Type A dietary recommendations. These foods are versatile and can be enjoyed in various ways, whether as snacks, in salads, or as ingredients in your favorite recipes.

# Oils and Fats

| Oil/Fat | Ingredients | Instructions | Nutritional Information (per serving) | Serving Size | Cooking Time |
|---|---|---|---|---|---|
| **Olive Oil** | 100% Extra Virgin Olive Oil | Use for salad dressings, drizzling over vegetables, or low-heat sautéing. | 120 calories, 14g fat (2g saturated fat), 0g carbs, 0g protein | 1 tablespoon | No cooking required |
| **Flaxseed Oil** | 100% Pure Flaxseed Oil | Add to smoothies, salads, or drizzled over cooked dishes. Do not heat. | 120 calories, 14g fat (1g saturated fat), 0g carbs, 0g protein | 1 tablespoon | No cooking required |

| Oil/Fat | Ingredients | Instructions | Nutritional Information (per serving) | Serving Size | Cooking Time |
|---|---|---|---|---|---|
| Walnut Oil | 100% Pure Walnut Oil | Use for salad dressings, drizzling over cooked vegetables or pasta. Do not heat. | 120 calories, 14g fat (1.5g saturated fat), 0g carbs, 0g protein | 1 tablespoon | No cooking required |
| Canola Oil | 100% Canola Oil | Use for baking, sautéing, or in salad dressings. | 120 calories, 14g fat (1g saturated fat), 0g carbs, 0g protein | 1 tablespoon | No cooking required |

| Oil/Fat | Ingredients | Instructions | Nutritional Information (per serving) | Serving Size | Cooking Time |
|---|---|---|---|---|---|
| **Hemp Seed Oil** | 100% Pure Hemp Seed Oil | Use for salad dressings or drizzling over dishes. Do not heat. | 120 calories, 14g fat (1g saturated fat), 0g carbs, 0g protein | 1 tablespoon | No cooking required |
| **Pumpkin Seed Oil** | 100% Pure Pumpkin Seed Oil | Use for salad dressings, drizzling over soups or vegetables. Do not heat. | 120 calories, 14g fat (2.5g saturated fat), 0g carbs, 0g protein | 1 tablespoon | No cooking required |
| **Sesame Oil** | 100% Pure Sesame Oil | Use for salad dressings or | 120 calories, 14g fat (2g | 1 tablespoon | No cooking required |

| Oil/Fat | Ingredients | Instructions | Nutritional Information (per serving) | Serving Size | Cooking Time |
|---|---|---|---|---|---|
|  |  | low-heat cooking. | saturated fat), 0g carbs, 0g protein |  |  |
| **Almond Oil** | 100% Pure Almond Oil | Use for baking, salad dressings, or drizzling over dishes. Do not heat. | 120 calories, 14g fat (1g saturated fat), 0g carbs, 0g protein | 1 tablespoon | No cooking required |
| **Avocado Oil** | 100% Pure Avocado Oil | Use for high-heat cooking, baking, or salad dressings. | 124 calories, 14g fat (2g saturated fat), 0g carbs, 0g protein | 1 tablespoon | No cooking required |

| Oil/Fat | Ingredients | Instructions | Nutritional Information (per serving) | Serving Size | Cooking Time |
|---|---|---|---|---|---|
| **Grapeseed Oil** | 100% Pure Grapeseed Oil | Use for baking, sautéing, or salad dressings. | 120 calories, 14g fat (1g saturated fat), 0g carbs, 0g protein | 1 tablespoon | No cooking required |
| **Sunflower Oil** | 100% Pure Sunflower Oil | Use for baking, sautéing, or salad dressings. | 120 calories, 14g fat (1.5g saturated fat), 0g carbs, 0g protein | 1 tablespoon | No cooking required |
| **Soybean Oil** | 100% Pure Soybean Oil | Use for baking, sautéing, or salad | 120 calories, 14g fat (2g saturated | 1 tablespoon | No cooking required |

| Oil/Fat | Ingredients | Instructions | Nutritional Information (per serving) | Serving Size | Cooking Time |
|---|---|---|---|---|---|
|  |  | dressings. | fat), 0g carbs, 0g protein |  |  |
| **Coconut Oil** | 100% Virgin Coconut Oil | Use for baking or medium-heat cooking. | 120 calories, 14g fat (12g saturated fat), 0g carbs, 0g protein | 1 tablespoon | No cooking required |
| **Macadamia Nut Oil** | 100% Pure Macadamia Nut Oil | Use for salad dressings or low-heat cooking. | 120 calories, 14g fat (2g saturated fat), 0g carbs, 0g protein | 1 tablespoon | No cooking required |

| Oil/Fat | Ingredients | Instructions | Nutritional Information (per serving) | Serving Size | Cooking Time |
| --- | --- | --- | --- | --- | --- |
| **Hazelnut Oil** | 100% Pure Hazelnut Oil | Use for salad dressings or drizzling over cooked dishes. Do not heat. | 120 calories, 14g fat (1g saturated fat), 0g carbs, 0g protein | 1 tablespoon | No cooking required |

**Olive Oil**: Known for its heart-healthy monounsaturated fats, olive oil is a staple in the Blood Type A diet. Use it to enhance the flavor of salads and cooked vegetables. With its antioxidants and anti-inflammatory properties, it supports overall health.

**Flaxseed Oil**: Rich in omega-3 fatty acids, flaxseed oil is an excellent addition to the diet for cardiovascular health and inflammation reduction. It should be used cold to preserve its nutritional benefits.

**Walnut Oil**: Another great source of omega-3 fatty acids, walnut oil adds a nutty flavor to dishes and supports brain health. It is best used in cold applications to maintain its nutrients.

**Canola Oil**: A versatile oil with a mild flavor, canola oil is low in saturated fat and high in heart-healthy monounsaturated fats. It can be used for a variety of cooking methods.

**Hemp Seed Oil**: This oil is rich in omega-3 and omega-6 fatty acids, promoting a balanced inflammatory response. Use it cold for salad dressings or finishing dishes.

**Pumpkin Seed Oil**: Known for its rich, nutty flavor and high antioxidant content, pumpkin seed oil supports prostate health and urinary function. Use it as a finishing oil for best results.

**Sesame Oil**: With its distinctive flavor, sesame oil is great for low-heat cooking and adding depth to dressings and marinades. It also contains beneficial lignans and antioxidants.

**Almond Oil**: Mild and slightly nutty, almond oil is excellent for dressings and drizzling over foods. It supports skin health due to its vitamin E content.

**Avocado Oil**: This oil is high in monounsaturated fats and has a high smoke point, making it suitable for high-heat cooking. It also supports eye and skin health.

**Grapeseed Oil**: Light and versatile, grapeseed oil is good for sautéing and baking. It contains vitamin E and antioxidants, promoting skin and heart health.

**Sunflower Oil**: With a mild flavor, sunflower oil is rich in vitamin E and low in saturated fat. It is suitable for various cooking methods, including baking and sautéing.

**Soybean Oil**: High in polyunsaturated fats, including omega-3 and omega-6 fatty acids, soybean oil supports cardiovascular health. Use it in dressings and for cooking.

**Coconut Oil**: Known for its medium-chain triglycerides (MCTs), coconut oil is suitable for medium-heat cooking and baking. It provides a quick source of energy and supports brain health.

**Macadamia Nut Oil**: This oil is rich in monounsaturated fats and has a buttery flavor. Use it for dressings or low-heat cooking to maintain its nutritional benefits.

**Hazelnut Oil**: With a rich, nutty flavor, hazelnut oil is excellent for cold applications like dressings and drizzling over finished dishes. It contains heart-healthy fats and antioxidants.

By incorporating these oils and fats into your diet, you can ensure that you are getting the essential fatty acids and nutrients necessary for optimal health and well-being, tailored specifically for Blood Type A.

# Proteins to Prioritize

| Protein | Ingredients | Instructions | Nutritional Information (per serving) | Serving Size | Cooking Time |
|---|---|---|---|---|---|
| Tofu | 1 block of firm tofu | Press tofu to remove excess water, cut into cubes, and bake at 375°F for 25 minutes. | 70 calories, 8g protein, 2g carbs, 4g fat | 1/4 block | 25 minutes |
| Tempeh | 1 package of tempeh | Slice tempeh, marinate in soy sauce and spices, and grill for 10 minutes per side. | 160 calories, 15g protein, 9g carbs, 8g fat | 1/2 package | 20 minutes |

| Protein | Ingredients | Instructions | Nutritional Information (per serving) | Serving Size | Cooking Time |
| --- | --- | --- | --- | --- | --- |
| Edamame | 1 cup of edamame (shelled) | Boil edamame in salted water for 5 minutes, then drain. | 120 calories, 11g protein, 10g carbs, 5g fat | 1 cup | 5 minutes |
| Lentils | 1 cup dried lentils | Rinse lentils, boil in water for 20 minutes until tender, and season with herbs. | 230 calories, 18g protein, 40g carbs, 1g fat | 1 cup cooked | 20 minutes |
| Chickpeas | 1 cup dried chickpeas | Soak overnight, boil in water for 45 minutes | 210 calories, 15g protein, 35g carbs, | 1 cup cooked | 45 minutes |

| Protein | Ingredients | Instructions | Nutritional Information (per serving) | Serving Size | Cooking Time |
|---|---|---|---|---|---|
| | | until soft, then season. | 3g fat | | |
| Black Beans | 1 cup dried black beans | Soak overnight, boil in water for 60 minutes until tender, then season. | 227 calories, 15g protein, 41g carbs, 1g fat | 1 cup cooked | 60 minutes |
| Quinoa | 1 cup quinoa | Rinse quinoa, cook in water for 15 minutes, fluff with a fork. | 222 calories, 8g protein, 39g carbs, 4g fat | 1 cup cooked | 15 minutes |

| Protein | Ingredients | Instructions | Nutritional Information (per serving) | Serving Size | Cooking Time |
| --- | --- | --- | --- | --- | --- |
| Pumpkin Seeds | 1/4 cup pumpkin seeds | Eat raw or toast in oven at 350°F for 10 minutes. | 180 calories, 7g protein, 15g carbs, 13g fat | 1/4 cup | 10 minutes |
| Almonds | 1/4 cup almonds | Eat raw or roast in oven at 350°F for 10 minutes. | 160 calories, 6g protein, 6g carbs, 14g fat | 1/4 cup | 10 minutes |
| Sunflower Seeds | 1/4 cup sunflower seeds | Eat raw or toast in oven at 350°F for 10 minutes. | 190 calories, 7g protein, 7g carbs, 16g fat | 1/4 cup | 10 minutes |
| Hemp Seeds | 3 tablespoons hemp | Sprinkle on salads or smoothies. | 170 calories, 10g | 3 tablespoons | None |

| Protein | Ingredients | Instructions | Nutritional Information (per serving) | Serving Size | Cooking Time |
| --- | --- | --- | --- | --- | --- |
|  | seeds | No cooking needed. | protein, 3g carbs, 13g fat |  |  |
| Chia Seeds | 2 tablespoons chia seeds | Mix in water or add to smoothies. No cooking needed. | 138 calories, 4g protein, 12g carbs, 9g fat | 2 tablespoons | None |
| Flaxseeds | 2 tablespoons flaxseeds | Grind and add to oatmeal or smoothies. No cooking needed. | 110 calories, 4g protein, 8g carbs, 8g fat | 2 tablespoons | None |
| Mung Beans | 1 cup dried mung beans | Soak overnight, boil in | 212 calories, 14g | 1 cup cooked | 30 minutes |

| Protein | Ingredients | Instructions | Nutritional Information (per serving) | Serving Size | Cooking Time |
|---|---|---|---|---|---|
| | | water for 30 minutes until tender, then season. | protein, 38g carbs, 1g fat | | |
| Spirulina | 1 tablespoon spirulina powder | Add to smoothies or juices. No cooking needed. | 20 calories, 4g protein, 2g carbs, 0.5g fat | 1 tablespoon | None |

Each of these proteins offers a range of nutritional benefits tailored to the needs of Blood Type A individuals. By incorporating these proteins into your diet, you can ensure a balanced intake of essential nutrients, supporting overall health and well-being.

# Foods to Avoid

## Meat and Poultry

| Food | Description | Reason to Avoid |
| --- | --- | --- |
| Beef | Includes cuts like steak, ground beef, and roasts. | Beef is high in saturated fats and cholesterol, which can contribute to cardiovascular issues and inflammation. Blood Type A individuals often have lower stomach acid, making it difficult to digest red meat efficiently. |
| Pork | Includes bacon, ham, pork chops, and sausages. | Pork is rich in saturated fats and cholesterol, which can lead to weight gain and heart disease. Additionally, it contains toxins and parasites that can be hard for Blood Type A individuals to process. |
| Lamb | Includes lamb chops, leg of lamb, and ground lamb. | Similar to beef, lamb is high in saturated fats and can be challenging for Blood Type A individuals to digest. It can also contribute to |

| Food | Description | Reason to Avoid |
|---|---|---|
| | | increased inflammation and digestive discomfort. |
| Veal | Includes veal cutlets, veal chops, and ground veal. | Veal is a form of red meat that can cause digestive strain and inflammation in Blood Type A individuals due to its high protein and fat content. |
| Venison | Includes deer meat, such as steaks and ground venison. | Although leaner than other red meats, venison still contains high levels of protein that can be difficult for Blood Type A to digest, potentially leading to digestive issues. |
| Duck | Includes duck breast, duck legs, and whole duck. | Duck meat is high in fat, particularly saturated fats, which can be problematic for Blood Type A. It can also be harder to digest and contribute to weight gain. |
| Goose | Includes goose breast, goose legs, and whole goose. | Similar to duck, goose meat is rich in fats that can lead to cardiovascular problems and are difficult for Blood Type A individuals to digest. |

| Food | Description | Reason to Avoid |
|---|---|---|
| **Rabbit** | Includes rabbit stew, roasted rabbit, and ground rabbit. | Rabbit meat, though lean, is still high in protein and can cause digestive difficulties for Blood Type A individuals, leading to potential discomfort and inflammation. |
| **Turkey** | Includes turkey breast, ground turkey, and turkey legs. | While leaner than other poultry, turkey can still be problematic for Blood Type A due to its potential to cause digestive issues and inflammation. |
| **Chicken** | Includes chicken breast, thighs, wings, and ground chicken. | Chicken is a common allergen and can be harder to digest for Blood Type A individuals, leading to potential digestive discomfort and inflammation. |
| **Quail** | Includes whole quail and quail breast. | Quail meat, similar to other poultry, can cause digestive issues and is high in protein that may be difficult for Blood Type A individuals to process efficiently. |
| **Cornish Hen** | Includes whole Cornish hen and | Cornish hen, being a form of poultry, can contribute to digestive strain and |

| Food | Description | Reason to Avoid |
| --- | --- | --- |
|  | Cornish hen parts. | inflammation in Blood Type A individuals due to its protein content. |
| **Pheasant** | Includes pheasant breast, legs, and whole pheasant. | Pheasant meat, though lean, can still cause digestive problems and inflammation for Blood Type A individuals due to its protein structure. |
| **Partridge** | Includes partridge breast, legs, and whole partridge. | Partridge meat, similar to other game birds, can be difficult for Blood Type A individuals to digest and may contribute to inflammation and digestive discomfort. |
| **Ostrich** | Includes ostrich steak, ground ostrich, and ostrich burgers. | Despite being a lean red meat, ostrich is still high in protein that can be hard for Blood Type A individuals to digest, potentially leading to inflammation and digestive issues. |

Avoiding these meats and poultry helps Blood Type A individuals maintain better digestive health and reduce inflammation. Instead, it is recommended to focus on plant-based proteins and seafood that are more easily digested and beneficial for their overall well-being. By making these dietary adjustments, individuals with Blood Type A can experience improved health outcomes and enhanced energy levels.

# Dairy Products

| Dairy Product | Reason to Avoid | Potential Health Effects |
|---|---|---|
| Whole Milk | High in saturated fats and difficult to digest due to low stomach acid levels in Blood Type A individuals | Bloating, digestive discomfort, increased mucus production |
| Cheese (Cheddar, Swiss, Brie, etc.) | High in saturated fats and lactose, which can cause digestive issues | Bloating, constipation, gas, potential lactose intolerance symptoms |
| Cream | High-fat content can be difficult to digest and can contribute to inflammation | Digestive issues, increased cholesterol levels, inflammation |
| Ice Cream | Contains high levels of sugar and lactose, leading to digestive disturbances and weight gain | Bloating, weight gain, blood sugar spikes |

| Dairy Product | Reason to Avoid | Potential Health Effects |
| --- | --- | --- |
| Butter | High in saturated fats and can lead to increased cholesterol and digestive issues | Increased cholesterol, potential heart health concerns, digestive discomfort |
| Yogurt | Though fermented, it still contains lactose and can cause digestive problems | Bloating, gas, potential lactose intolerance symptoms |
| Sour Cream | High in fat and lactose, which can be hard to digest | Digestive discomfort, increased mucus production, inflammation |
| Cottage Cheese | Contains lactose and casein, both of which can cause issues for Blood Type A individuals | Bloating, digestive discomfort, potential lactose intolerance symptoms |
| Cream Cheese | High in fat and lactose, leading to digestive issues and weight gain | Digestive discomfort, weight gain, increased |

| Dairy Product | Reason to Avoid | Potential Health Effects |
| --- | --- | --- |
| | | cholesterol levels |
| Ricotta Cheese | Contains lactose and can cause digestive problems for those with lower stomach acid | Bloating, gas, potential lactose intolerance symptoms |
| Mozzarella | Contains lactose and is high in fat, making it difficult to digest | Digestive issues, bloating, potential lactose intolerance symptoms |
| Feta Cheese | Though lower in fat, it still contains lactose and can cause issues | Bloating, digestive discomfort, potential lactose intolerance symptoms |
| Parmesan Cheese | Aged cheese but still contains lactose and can be difficult to digest | Digestive discomfort, bloating, increased cholesterol levels |
| Milk-based Soups and Sauces | High in lactose and fat, which can be hard to digest and cause inflammation | Digestive issues, increased mucus production, inflammation |

| Dairy Product | Reason to Avoid | Potential Health Effects |
| --- | --- | --- |
| Processed Dairy Products (e.g., Processed Cheese, Cheese Spreads) | Often contain additives and preservatives along with high levels of lactose and fats | Digestive discomfort, inflammation, potential adverse reactions to additives |

**Why Blood Type A Individuals Should Avoid Dairy Products**

**Digestive Discomfort**: Blood Type A individuals typically have lower levels of stomach acid, making it difficult to break down and digest the proteins and fats in dairy products. This can lead to symptoms such as bloating, gas, and abdominal discomfort.

**Increased Mucus Production**: Dairy products can increase mucus production, which can exacerbate respiratory issues and contribute to conditions such as asthma and sinusitis.

**Inflammation**: The high levels of saturated fats found in many dairy products can contribute to inflammation in the body. Chronic inflammation is linked to various health issues, including heart disease and arthritis.

**Lactose Intolerance**: Many people with Blood Type A have lactose intolerance to some degree. This means their bodies have difficulty breaking down lactose, the sugar found in milk, leading to symptoms like bloating, diarrhea, and gas.

**Cholesterol and Heart Health**: High-fat dairy products can increase cholesterol levels, which is a risk factor for heart disease. Blood Type A individuals are advised to focus on heart-healthy, low-fat, and plant-based alternatives.

**Weight Management**: Dairy products, especially those high in fat and sugar like ice cream, can contribute to weight gain. Managing weight is easier with a diet rich in plant-based proteins, fruits, and vegetables.

By avoiding these dairy products, Blood Type A individuals can improve their digestion, reduce inflammation, and support overall health. Instead, they should focus on plant-based alternatives like almond milk, soy milk, and coconut yogurt, which are easier to digest and provide essential nutrients without the adverse effects of dairy.

# Wheat and Gluten

| Food | Description | Reasons to Avoid |
| --- | --- | --- |
| **Wheat Bread** | Made from wheat flour, commonly used for sandwiches and toast. | Contains gluten which can cause digestive issues and inflammation in Blood Type A individuals. |
| **Pasta** | Traditional pasta is made from durum wheat. | High in gluten, which can lead to bloating and discomfort. |
| **Couscous** | Made from semolina wheat, often used in Mediterranean dishes. | Contains gluten, which can cause gastrointestinal distress and interfere with nutrient absorption. |
| **Wheat Bran** | Outer layer of the wheat kernel, often used in cereals and baked goods. | High in gluten, which can irritate the gut lining and lead to inflammation. |
| **Bulgur Wheat** | Whole grain made from cracked wheat, commonly used in Middle Eastern cuisine. | Contains gluten, which can trigger digestive issues and reduce overall well-being for Blood Type A. |

| Food | Description | Reasons to Avoid |
| --- | --- | --- |
| **Crackers** | Often made from wheat flour, used as snacks or with dips. | High in gluten, which can cause inflammation and digestive discomfort. |
| **Cakes and Pastries** | Typically made with wheat flour and often contain high amounts of sugar. | High in gluten and refined sugars, which can disrupt digestion and lead to weight gain. |
| **Cookies** | Made from wheat flour and usually high in sugar. | Contains gluten and refined sugars, which can cause bloating and blood sugar spikes. |
| **Pretzels** | Made from wheat flour, often consumed as snacks. | High in gluten, which can lead to digestive issues and inflammation. |
| **Beer** | Brewed from barley, wheat, and other grains, contains gluten. | Contains gluten, which can cause bloating and digestive discomfort. |
| **Barley** | A cereal grain used in soups, stews, and as a malt source for beverages. | Contains gluten, which can be difficult to digest for Blood Type A individuals. |
| **Rye** | Grain used in bread, | Contains gluten, which can |

| Food | Description | Reasons to Avoid |
|---|---|---|
| | crackers, and some alcoholic beverages. | cause digestive problems and inflammation. |
| Spelt | An ancient grain similar to wheat, used in baking and cooking. | High in gluten, which can trigger digestive issues and inflammation. |
| Seitan | A meat substitute made from wheat gluten, often used in vegetarian dishes. | Extremely high in gluten, which can cause significant digestive issues for Blood Type A individuals. |
| Farina | Milled wheat used to make hot cereal, also known as cream of wheat. | Contains gluten, which can cause bloating, discomfort, and inflammation. |

**Why You Should Avoid Wheat and Gluten**

1. **Digestive Issues:** Gluten can be difficult to digest, especially for individuals with Blood Type A, who tend to have a more sensitive digestive system. Consuming gluten can lead to bloating, gas, and discomfort.

2. **Inflammation:** Gluten can cause inflammation in the gut, which can lead to a range of health issues including leaky gut syndrome. This inflammation can exacerbate other conditions and reduce overall health.

3. **Nutrient Absorption:** The presence of gluten can interfere with the absorption of essential nutrients, leading to deficiencies over time. This is particularly concerning for Blood Type A individuals who need a nutrient-rich diet to support their immune system and overall health.

4. **Immune Response:** Gluten can trigger an immune response in some individuals, leading to symptoms such as fatigue, joint pain, and headaches. For Blood Type A, who already have a predisposition to immune-related issues, avoiding gluten can help maintain a balanced and strong immune system.

5. **Energy Levels:** Many people report feeling more energetic and less sluggish when they eliminate gluten from their diet. For Blood Type A individuals, who thrive on a plant-based diet, removing gluten can help maintain consistent energy levels throughout the day.

By avoiding these wheat and gluten-containing foods, Blood Type A individuals can improve their digestive health, reduce inflammation, and enhance their overall well-being. Instead, focus on incorporating gluten-free grains and other suitable alternatives to maintain a balanced and nutritious diet.

# Certain Vegetables and Fruits

| Vegetable/Fruit | Reason to Avoid |
| --- | --- |
| **Tomatoes** | Contain lectins that can irritate the stomach lining and lead to digestive issues. |
| **Potatoes** | High in lectins that may disrupt gastrointestinal health and contribute to inflammation. |
| **Cabbage** | Contains compounds that can interfere with thyroid function, which is a common issue for Blood Type A individuals. |
| **Peppers** | Both sweet and hot peppers can cause stomach irritation and exacerbate acid reflux in Blood Type A individuals. |
| **Eggplant** | Contains lectins that can irritate the stomach lining and cause digestive discomfort. |
| **Mushrooms** | Certain types of mushrooms can be difficult to digest and may cause digestive issues. |
| **Olives** | Often preserved in brine, which can cause inflammation and water retention in Blood Type A individuals. |
| **Oranges** | Highly acidic and can contribute to stomach irritation and digestive issues. |

| Vegetable/Fruit | Reason to Avoid |
| --- | --- |
| Bananas | Can disrupt blood sugar levels and are harder to digest for Blood Type A individuals. |
| Mangoes | High in sugar and can cause digestive issues and blood sugar spikes. |
| Papayas | Can disrupt digestive balance and cause discomfort due to their high enzyme content. |
| Coconut | Contains saturated fats that are harder for Blood Type A individuals to digest and can affect cholesterol levels. |
| Tangerines | Highly acidic and can cause digestive issues similar to oranges. |
| Melons | Can cause digestive discomfort and bloating due to their high water content and sugars. |
| Avocados | High in fats that may be harder for Blood Type A individuals to digest and can cause digestive issues. |

**Explanation of Why to Avoid These Foods**

**Tomatoes and Potatoes:** These vegetables contain high levels of lectins, which are proteins that can bind to the gut lining and cause irritation and inflammation. This can lead to digestive issues and exacerbate existing conditions.

**Cabbage:** This vegetable contains goitrogens, which are substances that can interfere with thyroid function. Since Blood Type A individuals are more prone to thyroid issues, avoiding cabbage helps prevent potential complications.

**Peppers (Sweet and Hot):** Peppers contain capsaicin and other compounds that can irritate the stomach lining, leading to discomfort and potential exacerbation of acid reflux.

**Eggplant:** Similar to tomatoes and peppers, eggplant contains lectins that can irritate the digestive tract and cause discomfort.

**Mushrooms:** Certain types of mushrooms can be hard to digest and may cause bloating and other digestive issues for Blood Type A individuals.

**Olives:** Often preserved in brine, olives can lead to inflammation and water retention, which are detrimental to Blood Type A individuals who are prone to these issues.

**Oranges, Tangerines, and Other Citrus Fruits:** These fruits are highly acidic and can cause stomach irritation and digestive issues, particularly for those with a sensitive digestive system like Blood Type A individuals.

**Bananas and Mangoes:** These fruits are high in sugar, which can disrupt blood sugar levels and cause digestive discomfort. They may also lead to bloating and other gastrointestinal issues.

**Papayas:** While generally nutritious, papayas contain high levels of enzymes that can disrupt digestive balance and cause discomfort in some Blood Type A individuals.

**Coconut:** Contains saturated fats that are more challenging for Blood Type A individuals to digest, potentially affecting cholesterol levels and causing digestive issues.

**Melons:** High water content and sugars in melons can lead to digestive discomfort, bloating, and upset stomach in Blood Type A individuals.

**Avocados:** Though healthy for many, avocados are high in fats that may be harder for Blood Type A individuals to digest, leading to potential digestive issues and discomfort.

By avoiding these vegetables and fruits, Blood Type A individuals can better manage their digestive health and overall well-being. Adjusting the diet to exclude these items can help prevent inflammation, digestive discomfort, and other adverse reactions.

# Unfavorable Beans and Legumes

| Bean/Legume | Reason to Avoid |
| --- | --- |
| **Kidney Beans** | Kidney beans contain lectins that can cause digestive distress and interfere with nutrient absorption for Blood Type A individuals. These lectins can bind to the intestinal lining, potentially leading to inflammation and gastrointestinal issues. |
| **Lima Beans** | Lima beans have high levels of certain lectins that can disrupt the digestive system of Blood Type A individuals. Consuming lima beans may lead to symptoms such as bloating, gas, and abdominal discomfort. |
| **Navy Beans** | Navy beans contain lectins that are not well tolerated by Blood Type A individuals. These lectins can cause inflammation in the gut and impair the digestion and absorption of other nutrients. |

| Bean/Legume | Reason to Avoid |
| --- | --- |
| **Red Beans** | Similar to kidney beans, red beans are high in lectins that can cause digestive problems for Blood Type A. These lectins can trigger immune responses and inflammation in the digestive tract. |
| **Black-eyed Peas** | Black-eyed peas contain lectins that can adversely affect Blood Type A individuals. These lectins can cause digestive issues and may contribute to inflammation in the intestines. |
| **Garbanzos (Chickpeas)** | Chickpeas contain lectins that can be problematic for Blood Type A. These lectins may cause gastrointestinal discomfort and interfere with nutrient assimilation. |
| **Fava Beans** | Fava beans are high in lectins that are particularly hard on the digestive system of Blood Type A individuals. Consuming fava beans can lead to digestive disturbances and potential inflammation. |
| **Cranberry Beans** | Cranberry beans contain lectins that can cause adverse reactions in Blood Type A |

| Bean/Legume | Reason to Avoid |
| --- | --- |
|  | individuals. These lectins may lead to bloating, gas, and discomfort in the digestive system. |
| Pinto Beans | Pinto beans are another legume with high lectin content that can negatively impact the digestion of Blood Type A individuals. These lectins can cause digestive distress and inflammation. |
| Soybeans (in certain forms) | While some fermented soy products like tempeh are beneficial, whole soybeans and unfermented soy products contain lectins that can disrupt digestion for Blood Type A. Unfermented soy can cause bloating, gas, and interfere with nutrient absorption. |
| Peanuts | Although not a legume, peanuts are often grouped with beans and legumes. Peanuts contain lectins and allergens that can cause significant digestive issues and inflammatory responses in Blood Type A individuals. |
| Adzuki Beans | Adzuki beans contain lectins that can |

| Bean/Legume | Reason to Avoid |
| --- | --- |
|  | cause digestive problems for Blood Type A. These lectins can lead to gastrointestinal discomfort and interfere with proper digestion. |
| Black Beans | Black beans are high in lectins that can be problematic for Blood Type A individuals. These lectins can cause inflammation and digestive issues. |
| Cannellini Beans | Cannellini beans, like other legumes high in lectins, can disrupt digestion for Blood Type A individuals. Consuming these beans can lead to symptoms such as bloating and gastrointestinal discomfort. |
| Mung Beans | Mung beans, despite their nutrient profile, contain lectins that can cause digestive issues for Blood Type A. These lectins can trigger inflammation and digestive discomfort. |

| Nuts/Seeds | Why You Should Avoid It |
| --- | --- |
| Cashews | Cashews contain lectins that can interfere with digestive enzymes and cause inflammation in the digestive tract. They may also contribute to weight gain and joint pain for individuals with Blood Type A. |
| Pistachios | Pistachios can cause digestive issues and bloating due to their high lectin content. They may also lead to an imbalance in the gut flora, which is crucial for Blood Type A individuals who need a healthy digestive system. |
| Brazil Nuts | Brazil nuts are high in saturated fats, which can be difficult for Blood Type A individuals to digest and may lead to weight gain and cardiovascular issues. They also contain lectins that can cause inflammation. |
| Macadamia Nuts | Macadamia nuts are high in fat and can be hard to digest, leading to digestive discomfort and weight gain. Their lectin content can also cause inflammation in Blood Type A individuals. |
| Peanuts | Peanuts contain high levels of lectins and |

| Nuts/Seeds | Why You Should Avoid It |
| --- | --- |
|  | aflatoxins, which can disrupt digestion and cause inflammation. They may also contribute to an increased risk of heart disease and cancer in Blood Type A individuals. |
| **Hazelnuts** | Hazelnuts can be difficult for Blood Type A individuals to digest and may cause bloating and gas. They also contain lectins that can interfere with the absorption of other nutrients. |
| **Sesame Seeds** | Sesame seeds contain lectins that can irritate the digestive tract and cause inflammation. They may also lead to allergic reactions and should be avoided by Blood Type A individuals. |
| **Sunflower Seeds** | Sunflower seeds can cause digestive issues and inflammation due to their high lectin content. They may also interfere with the absorption of essential nutrients and cause allergic reactions in some Blood Type A individuals. |
| **Pumpkin Seeds** | While beneficial for other blood types, pumpkin seeds can cause digestive discomfort and inflammation in Blood Type A individuals due to their lectin content. They may also contribute to allergic reactions. |

| Nuts/Seeds | Why You Should Avoid It |
| --- | --- |
| Pine Nuts | Pine nuts can be hard to digest and may cause bloating and digestive discomfort for Blood Type A individuals. They also contain lectins that can interfere with nutrient absorption and cause inflammation. |
| Walnuts | Walnuts contain high levels of omega-6 fatty acids, which can cause inflammation and imbalance in the fatty acid profile of Blood Type A individuals. They can also be difficult to digest and lead to digestive issues. |
| Pecans | Pecans are high in fat and can be difficult for Blood Type A individuals to digest. They may cause digestive discomfort and weight gain, as well as inflammation due to their lectin content. |
| Chia Seeds | Chia seeds can cause digestive issues and bloating for Blood Type A individuals due to their high fiber content and lectins. They may also lead to allergic reactions and should be consumed with caution. |
| Flaxseeds | Flaxseeds contain high levels of phytoestrogens and lectins, which can interfere with hormone balance and cause inflammation in Blood Type A |

| Nuts/Seeds | Why You Should Avoid It |
|---|---|
|  | individuals. They can also lead to digestive discomfort. |
| **Hemp Seeds** | Hemp seeds can cause digestive issues and bloating for Blood Type A individuals due to their high fiber content and lectins. They may also interfere with nutrient absorption and cause allergic reactions. |

By avoiding these unfavorable nuts and seeds, Blood Type A individuals can prevent digestive discomfort, inflammation, and other health issues. It is important to focus on foods that align with their specific nutritional needs to maintain optimal health and well-being.

# Harmful Oils and Fats

| Harmful Oil/Fat | Reason to Avoid |
|---|---|
| **Corn Oil** | Corn oil is high in omega-6 fatty acids, which can promote inflammation in the body. For Blood Type A individuals, this inflammation can lead to digestive issues and a weakened immune system. |
| **Cottonseed Oil** | Cottonseed oil often contains high levels of pesticides and is heavily processed. It also has a poor fatty acid profile that can disrupt the balance of omega-3 and omega-6 fatty acids, leading to inflammation and other health issues. |
| **Canola Oil** | While canola oil is often marketed as a healthy option, it is highly processed and can contain trans fats, which are harmful to heart health. Blood Type A individuals may experience adverse effects on cardiovascular health and increased inflammation. |
| **Safflower Oil** | Safflower oil is another oil high in omega-6 fatty acids. Excessive intake can lead to an imbalance in the body's fatty acid profile, promoting inflammation and exacerbating health issues common in Blood Type A individuals, such as |

| Harmful Oil/Fat | Reason to Avoid |
| --- | --- |
| | digestive problems and immune system challenges. |
| **Peanut Oil** | Peanut oil contains a high amount of omega-6 fatty acids and can cause inflammation. Additionally, peanuts can be difficult for Blood Type A individuals to digest, potentially leading to gastrointestinal distress. |
| **Palm Oil** | Palm oil is high in saturated fats, which can increase cholesterol levels and contribute to heart disease. Blood Type A individuals should avoid it to maintain heart health and reduce the risk of inflammatory conditions. |
| **Soybean Oil** | Soybean oil is prevalent in processed foods and is high in omega-6 fatty acids, which can promote inflammation. For Blood Type A individuals, consuming soybean oil can lead to digestive issues and negatively impact overall health. |
| **Shortening** | Shortening contains trans fats, which are detrimental to cardiovascular health. For Blood Type A individuals, these fats can lead to increased |

| Harmful Oil/Fat | Reason to Avoid |
| --- | --- |
|  | inflammation, digestive issues, and a higher risk of chronic diseases. |
| Margarine | Margarine often contains trans fats and artificial additives. These components can disrupt heart health and promote inflammation, which are particularly harmful to Blood Type A individuals. |
| Hydrogenated Oils | Hydrogenated oils are used in many processed foods and contain trans fats, which are extremely harmful. They can increase the risk of heart disease and inflammation, making them particularly dangerous for Blood Type A individuals. |
| Lard | Lard is high in saturated fats, which can raise cholesterol levels and promote heart disease. Blood Type A individuals should avoid it to protect cardiovascular health and reduce inflammation. |
| Butter | Butter is high in saturated fats and can be difficult for Blood Type A individuals to digest. It can also contribute to high cholesterol levels and heart disease, making it a less suitable fat option. |
| Coconut Oil | Despite its popularity, coconut oil is high in saturated fats. For Blood Type A individuals, it can |

| Harmful Oil/Fat | Reason to Avoid |
| --- | --- |
| | contribute to elevated cholesterol levels and inflammation, which are detrimental to heart health and overall well-being. |
| Sunflower Oil | Sunflower oil is high in omega-6 fatty acids, which can cause inflammation when consumed in excess. For Blood Type A individuals, this can exacerbate digestive issues and other inflammatory conditions. |
| Grapeseed Oil | Grapeseed oil, though high in polyunsaturated fats, contains a high amount of omega-6 fatty acids. Excessive intake can lead to an imbalance and promote inflammation, which is not ideal for Blood Type A individuals. |

By avoiding these harmful oils and fats, individuals with Blood Type A can reduce inflammation, improve digestive health, and support overall wellness. Opting for healthier fats such as olive oil, flaxseed oil, and avocado oil can provide essential nutrients without the negative side effects associated with the oils and fats listed above.

# Essential Supplements

## Recommended Vitamins and Minerals

For individuals with Blood Type A, focusing on essential vitamins and minerals is crucial for maintaining optimal health. These nutrients play vital roles in supporting the immune system, enhancing energy levels, and promoting overall well-being. Including specific vitamins and minerals in your diet can help address any nutritional gaps and improve your health outcomes.

Vitamin A is important for immune function, vision, and skin health. Blood Type A individuals should prioritize sources of beta-carotene, which the body converts to vitamin A. Foods like carrots, sweet potatoes, and dark leafy greens such as spinach and kale are excellent choices. These foods provide the necessary nutrients while supporting the body's immune response and skin integrity.

Vitamin C is known for its immune-boosting properties and its role in collagen synthesis. Blood Type A individuals should include fruits and vegetables high in vitamin C, such as strawberries, oranges, and bell peppers. These foods help enhance immune function and promote healthy skin and tissues.

Vitamin D is essential for bone health and immune function. Since Blood Type A individuals may avoid dairy, which is a common source of vitamin D, they should seek alternative sources. Fortified plant-based milk, such as almond milk or soy milk, and exposure to sunlight are good ways to ensure adequate vitamin D levels. Additionally, supplements can be considered if natural sources are insufficient.

Vitamin E acts as an antioxidant, protecting cells from damage and supporting immune function. Nuts and seeds, such as almonds and sunflower seeds, are rich in vitamin E and are suitable for Blood Type A individuals. Including these foods in your diet can help maintain healthy skin and support the immune system.

Folate is critical for DNA synthesis and repair. Blood Type A individuals should consume leafy green vegetables like spinach, romaine lettuce, and legumes such as lentils and chickpeas. These foods are excellent sources of folate and can help prevent deficiencies that might otherwise lead to health complications.

Vitamin B12 is essential for red blood cell formation and neurological function. Since Blood Type A individuals may follow a more plant-based diet, they might need to consider fortified foods or supplements to meet their vitamin B12 needs. Fortified cereals, nutritional yeast, and supplements can help ensure adequate intake.

Iron is necessary for oxygen transport and energy production. Blood Type A individuals can obtain iron from plant-based sources like spinach, lentils, and tofu. To enhance iron absorption, it is beneficial to pair these foods with vitamin C-rich foods. This combination helps improve iron bioavailability and supports overall energy levels.

Calcium is crucial for bone health and muscle function. Since dairy products are not typically recommended for Blood Type A individuals, they should focus on plant-based sources of calcium. Leafy greens like kale and broccoli, as well as fortified plant-based milk alternatives, can provide adequate calcium to support bone health.

Magnesium plays a role in muscle and nerve function, blood sugar regulation, and bone health. Nuts and seeds, such as almonds and flaxseeds, along with whole grains like quinoa, are rich in magnesium. Including these foods in your diet helps ensure you get enough magnesium for various bodily functions.

Zinc is vital for immune function, wound healing, and protein synthesis. Blood Type A individuals can obtain zinc from plant-based sources like pumpkin seeds, sesame seeds, and chickpeas. These foods provide the necessary zinc without the need for animal products that may not align with the Blood Type A dietary guidelines.

Omega-3 fatty acids are important for heart health, reducing inflammation, and supporting brain function. Blood Type A individuals are encouraged to consume fish like salmon and mackerel. For those following a vegetarian or vegan diet, chia seeds, flaxseeds, and walnuts are excellent plant-based sources of omega-3 fatty acids.

Iodine is essential for thyroid function and metabolism. Sea vegetables such as nori, kelp, and dulse are excellent sources of iodine and can be easily incorporated into a Blood Type A diet. Ensuring adequate iodine intake helps maintain a healthy thyroid and supports metabolic processes.

Selenium is important for immune function and acts as an antioxidant. Brazil nuts are a particularly rich source of selenium and can be included in the diet to ensure adequate intake. Including just a few Brazil nuts in your diet can provide the necessary selenium for overall health.

By focusing on these recommended vitamins and minerals and incorporating the suggested foods into your diet, Blood Type A individuals can achieve a balanced intake of essential nutrients. This approach supports overall health, enhances immune function, and promotes optimal bodily functions.

# Importance of Supplementation

For individuals with Blood Type A, supplementation can play a crucial role in ensuring optimal health and well-being. While a well-balanced diet provides the foundation for good health, certain nutrients may still be lacking due to dietary restrictions or individual nutritional needs. Supplementation helps fill these gaps, supporting various bodily functions and enhancing overall health.

Vitamin B12 is particularly important for Blood Type A individuals, as this group often follows a vegetarian or low-meat diet. Vitamin B12 is essential for red blood cell formation, neurological function, and DNA synthesis. Since it is primarily found in animal products, supplementation with a high-quality B12 supplement can prevent deficiencies that may lead to anemia, fatigue, and cognitive issues.

Folic acid, or folate, is another vital nutrient for Blood Type A individuals. It supports DNA synthesis, repair, and cell division, playing a critical role in maintaining healthy blood cells. Folate is naturally present in leafy green vegetables, legumes, and some fruits. However, supplementation may be necessary to ensure adequate intake, especially for those with increased needs such as pregnant women.

Iron is essential for oxygen transport and energy production. Blood Type A individuals who avoid red meat may be at risk of iron deficiency. Plant-based sources of iron, such as spinach and lentils, provide non-heme iron, which is less readily absorbed by the body compared to heme iron found in animal products. Supplementing with iron can help prevent anemia, fatigue, and weakened immunity.

Vitamin D is crucial for bone health, immune function, and inflammation reduction. Blood Type A individuals, particularly those living in areas with limited sunlight exposure, may be at risk of vitamin D deficiency. A vitamin D supplement can support bone density, reduce the risk of fractures, and enhance immune response.

Omega-3 fatty acids are important for cardiovascular health, reducing inflammation, and supporting brain function. Blood Type A individuals who avoid fatty fish may not get enough omega-3s from their diet. Supplementation with fish oil or algae-based omega-3 supplements can help maintain heart health, support cognitive function, and reduce inflammation.

Calcium is necessary for bone health, nerve transmission, and muscle function. Blood Type A individuals who avoid dairy products need to ensure they get enough calcium from other sources. While leafy greens and fortified plant-based milks provide some calcium, supplementation may be necessary to prevent deficiencies that could lead to osteoporosis and other bone-related issues.



Magnesium is involved in over 300 enzymatic reactions in the body, including energy production, muscle function, and nerve transmission. Blood Type A individuals can benefit from magnesium supplementation, especially if their diet lacks sufficient amounts from nuts, seeds, and whole grains. Magnesium supplements can help reduce muscle cramps, support heart health, and improve sleep quality.

Zinc is essential for immune function, wound healing, and protein synthesis. Blood Type A individuals, particularly those on a vegetarian diet, may not get enough zinc from their food alone. Supplementation with zinc can enhance immune response, support skin health, and aid in proper growth and development.

Probiotics are beneficial for gut health, which is particularly important for Blood Type A individuals who may have sensitive digestive systems. Probiotic supplements can help maintain a healthy balance of gut bacteria, improve digestion, and boost the immune system.

Vitamin C is crucial for immune support, collagen synthesis, and antioxidant protection. While Blood Type A individuals can get vitamin C from fruits and vegetables, supplementation may be beneficial during times of increased stress or illness to ensure adequate intake and support overall health.

Supplementation tailored to the specific needs of Blood Type A individuals helps bridge nutritional gaps, supporting optimal health and well-being. By focusing on these essential nutrients, individuals can enhance their diet, prevent deficiencies, and promote long-term health.

# How to Incorporate Supplements

For individuals with Blood Type A, incorporating supplements can play a vital role in ensuring optimal health and addressing specific nutritional needs. Supplements can help fill gaps in the diet, support immune function, and enhance overall well-being. Here are some essential supplements for Blood Type A and how to effectively incorporate them into your daily routine.

Vitamin B12 is crucial for blood formation and neurological function. Since Blood Type A individuals often follow a vegetarian or semi-vegetarian diet, they might lack sufficient B12. To incorporate this supplement, take a daily or weekly B12 tablet or sublingual drop. Ensure to follow the recommended dosage on the product label.

Vitamin D is essential for bone health, immune support, and mood regulation. Blood Type A individuals might be at risk of vitamin D deficiency, especially if they live in areas with limited sunlight. Taking a vitamin D supplement daily can help maintain adequate levels. Choose vitamin D3 for better absorption and follow the dosage recommendations based on your age and health needs.

Calcium is important for maintaining strong bones and teeth. While Blood Type A individuals are advised to avoid most dairy products, they can take a calcium supplement to meet their needs. Calcium citrate is a good option as it is easily absorbed. Take it with meals to enhance absorption and avoid taking it with high-iron foods to prevent interference with iron absorption.

Magnesium supports muscle and nerve function, blood sugar control, and bone health. Incorporate a magnesium supplement by taking it daily, preferably in the evening as it can also help with relaxation and sleep. Magnesium glycinate is a well-absorbed form that is gentle on the stomach.

Iron is essential for oxygen transport and energy production. Plant-based diets common among Blood Type A individuals may lack adequate iron. To incorporate an iron supplement, choose a gentle, non-constipating form such as ferrous bisglycinate. Take it with a source of vitamin C to enhance absorption and avoid taking it with calcium supplements as they can interfere with iron absorption.

Zinc supports immune function, wound healing, and protein synthesis. Blood Type A individuals can benefit from taking a zinc supplement, especially during cold and flu season. Zinc picolinate or zinc citrate are good options. Follow the recommended dosage and take it with food to avoid stomach upset.

Probiotics are beneficial for digestive health and immune function. To incorporate probiotics, choose a high-quality supplement with multiple strains of beneficial bacteria. Take it daily, preferably on an empty stomach or with a small amount of food, and consider rotating different probiotic strains periodically to maintain a diverse gut microbiome.

Omega-3 fatty acids support heart health, reduce inflammation, and enhance brain function. Blood Type A individuals can incorporate an omega-3 supplement derived from fish oil or algae oil. Take it with meals to improve absorption and reduce the likelihood of fishy aftertaste. Follow the dosage recommendations on the product label.

Folic acid is important for DNA synthesis and repair, especially for women of childbearing age. Blood Type A individuals can incorporate a folic acid supplement by taking it daily as part of a multivitamin or prenatal vitamin. Ensure to follow the recommended dosage, especially if you are pregnant or planning to become pregnant.

Iodine is essential for thyroid function and metabolic regulation. Blood Type A individuals can incorporate iodine by taking a supplement derived from kelp or a multivitamin that includes iodine. Follow the dosage recommendations and avoid excessive intake, as too much iodine can cause thyroid dysfunction.

Vitamin E is an antioxidant that supports immune function and skin health. To incorporate vitamin E, take a natural form of the supplement, such as d-alpha-tocopherol. Follow the dosage recommendations and consider taking it with meals that contain healthy fats to enhance absorption.

Coenzyme Q10 (CoQ10) supports heart health and energy production. Blood Type A individuals can incorporate CoQ10 by taking a daily supplement, especially if they are taking statin medications, which can deplete CoQ10 levels. Choose a form like ubiquinol for better absorption and take it with meals.

Turmeric is known for its anti-inflammatory and antioxidant properties. To incorporate turmeric, take a supplement that includes black pepper extract (piperine) to enhance absorption. Follow the recommended dosage and consider taking it with meals to reduce the risk of stomach upset.

Resveratrol is an antioxidant that supports heart health and longevity. Blood Type A individuals can incorporate resveratrol by taking a daily supplement derived from red grapes or Japanese knotweed. Follow the dosage recommendations and take it with meals for better absorption.

By incorporating these essential supplements into your daily routine, you can ensure that you are meeting your nutritional needs and supporting your overall health as a Blood Type A individual. Always consult with a healthcare professional before starting any new supplement regimen to tailor it to your specific health requirements.

# Herbal Remedies

## Beneficial Herbs for Blood Type A

For individuals with Blood Type A, incorporating beneficial herbs into their diet can provide numerous health benefits, including improved digestion, enhanced immune function, and reduced inflammation. Below is a detailed guide on the most beneficial herbs for Blood Type A and their specific advantages.

Turmeric is a powerful anti-inflammatory herb that can help reduce inflammation and support joint health. The active compound, curcumin, has antioxidant properties that boost the immune system and protect against chronic diseases. Turmeric can be added to curries, soups, and smoothies for a health boost.

Garlic is known for its immune-boosting properties and can help lower blood pressure and cholesterol levels. It also has antiviral and antibacterial effects, making it an excellent herb for enhancing overall health. Fresh garlic can be used in cooking or taken as a supplement.

Ginger aids in digestion and has anti-inflammatory and antioxidant properties. It can help alleviate nausea, reduce muscle pain, and improve cardiovascular health. Ginger can be used fresh in teas, smoothies, and stir-fries, or as a powdered spice in various dishes.

Parsley is rich in vitamins A, C, and K, and acts as a natural diuretic, helping to eliminate excess fluid and reduce bloating. It also supports kidney health and can help freshen breath. Parsley can be used as a garnish or added to salads, soups, and sauces.

Echinacea is well-known for its immune-boosting properties and can help reduce the duration and severity of colds and other infections. It also has anti-inflammatory effects. Echinacea can be taken as a tea, tincture, or in supplement form.

Peppermint aids digestion by relieving symptoms of indigestion, gas, and bloating. It has antispasmodic properties that can help relax the gastrointestinal tract. Peppermint can be consumed as a tea, added to water, or used in cooking.

Chamomile is calming and helps reduce stress and anxiety, promoting better sleep. It also has anti-inflammatory and antispasmodic properties that aid in digestion. Chamomile is most commonly consumed as a tea.

Licorice root has anti-inflammatory and immune-boosting properties and can help soothe gastrointestinal issues like ulcers and acid reflux. However, it should be used in moderation due to its potential side effects on blood pressure. Licorice root can be taken as a tea or in supplement form.

Rosemary enhances memory and concentration and has anti-inflammatory and antioxidant properties. It also supports digestive health and can help alleviate headaches. Rosemary can be used fresh or dried in cooking, particularly with roasted vegetables and meats.

Basil is rich in antioxidants and has anti-inflammatory, antimicrobial, and immune-boosting properties. It can help reduce oxidative stress and support cardiovascular health. Basil can be used fresh in salads, sauces, and as a garnish for various dishes.

Lemon balm helps reduce stress and anxiety, promotes sleep, and supports digestive health. It has antiviral properties and can help alleviate cold sores. Lemon balm is typically consumed as a tea.

Oregano is rich in antioxidants and has antimicrobial properties, which can help fight off infections. It also supports respiratory health and has anti-inflammatory effects. Oregano can be used fresh or dried in cooking, especially in Italian and Mediterranean dishes.

Thyme is packed with vitamins C and A and has antimicrobial and anti-inflammatory properties. It supports respiratory health and can help relieve coughs and bronchitis. Thyme can be used fresh or dried in cooking, particularly in soups, stews, and roasted dishes.

Dandelion root acts as a natural diuretic and supports liver health by aiding in detoxification. It also has anti-inflammatory and antioxidant properties. Dandelion root can be consumed as a tea or in supplement form.

Sage has antimicrobial and anti-inflammatory properties and can help improve memory and cognitive function. It also supports digestive health and can alleviate sore throats. Sage can be used fresh or dried in cooking, especially in poultry and stuffing recipes.

Incorporating these beneficial herbs into your diet can enhance the overall health and well-being of individuals with Blood Type A. They can be easily added to meals, consumed as teas, or taken in supplement form to provide a range of health benefits tailored to the unique needs of Blood Type A individuals.

# How to Use Herbs in Cooking

For individuals with Blood Type A, incorporating specific herbs into cooking can enhance flavor while also providing numerous health benefits. These herbs can help improve digestion, boost the immune system, and reduce inflammation, all of which are particularly important for Blood Type A individuals. Here are detailed guidelines on how to use various herbs in your cooking:

**Basil** is a versatile herb that can be used fresh or dried. It pairs well with tomatoes, making it an excellent addition to salads, sauces, and soups. Basil is known for its anti-inflammatory properties and can help with digestion. Add fresh basil leaves to a caprese salad, or stir chopped basil into pasta sauces and soups just before serving to preserve its flavor and nutritional benefits.

**Garlic** is a potent herb with antibacterial and antiviral properties. It can be used fresh, minced, or powdered. Garlic is beneficial for cardiovascular health and immune support. Sauté minced garlic in olive oil as a base for sauces and stir-fries, or roast whole garlic cloves and spread them on whole grain bread for a flavorful, health-boosting snack.

**Ginger** is a powerful anti-inflammatory herb that aids in digestion and helps alleviate nausea. Use fresh ginger by grating it into teas, smoothies, and marinades. Add sliced ginger to stir-fries and soups for a zesty kick. Ginger powder can also be used in baking or sprinkled into curry dishes.

**Turmeric** contains curcumin, which has strong anti-inflammatory and antioxidant properties. Use ground turmeric in curries, soups, and rice dishes. Turmeric can also be added to smoothies or golden milk for an anti-inflammatory boost. Combining turmeric with black pepper enhances the absorption of curcumin in the body.

**Parsley** is a fresh herb that can be used to garnish a variety of dishes. It is rich in vitamins A, C, and K and supports detoxification. Chop fresh parsley and sprinkle it over salads, soups, and grain dishes. Add parsley to homemade dressings and marinades for a burst of freshness.

**Rosemary** has a robust, pine-like flavor and is great for improving memory and concentration. Use fresh or dried rosemary to season roasted vegetables, meats, and potatoes. Infuse olive oil with rosemary sprigs for a flavorful cooking oil. Add rosemary to homemade bread dough for a fragrant and tasty loaf.

**Thyme** is an aromatic herb with antibacterial properties that supports respiratory health. Use fresh or dried thyme in soups, stews, and roasted dishes. Thyme pairs well with lemon and garlic, making it a great addition to marinades for poultry and fish. Sprinkle dried thyme into stuffing or casseroles for added depth of flavor.

**Oregano** is known for its antimicrobial and antioxidant properties. Use fresh or dried oregano in tomato-based dishes, salads, and Mediterranean recipes. Add oregano to homemade pizza, pasta sauces, and salad dressings. Sprinkle dried oregano over roasted vegetables or mix it into marinades for a robust flavor.

**Mint** is a refreshing herb that aids in digestion and soothes the stomach. Use fresh mint leaves in teas, salads, and desserts. Mint pairs well with fruits, especially berries and melons, and can be added to yogurt and smoothies. Make a refreshing mint-infused water or add mint leaves to lamb and other Mediterranean dishes.

**Cilantro** has a unique flavor and is known for its detoxifying properties. Use fresh cilantro leaves in salsas, salads, and soups. Add cilantro to guacamole, tacos, and rice dishes for a burst of flavor. Cilantro can also be blended into smoothies for a detoxifying drink.

**Sage** has a strong, earthy flavor and is known for its anti-inflammatory and antioxidant properties. Use fresh or dried sage in stuffing, sausages, and roasted dishes. Sage pairs well with poultry, pork, and root vegetables. Add sage to browned butter and drizzle over pasta or roasted squash.

**Dill** is a fresh herb that supports digestive health and has a mild, slightly tangy flavor. Use fresh dill in salads, soups, and seafood dishes. Add dill to yogurt-based dressings and sauces, or sprinkle it over roasted carrots and potatoes. Dill can also be used to flavor pickles and other preserved vegetables.

**Cilantro** (coriander leaves) is excellent for detoxification and supports healthy digestion. Use fresh cilantro in salsas, salads, and soups. Add cilantro to curries, rice dishes, and stir-fries for a burst of fresh flavor. Blend cilantro into green smoothies or use it to garnish tacos and burritos.

By incorporating these herbs into your cooking, you can enhance the flavors of your meals while also reaping the health benefits they offer. These herbs align well with the dietary needs of Blood Type A individuals and can contribute to a balanced and nutritious diet.

# Herbal Teas and Infusions

For individuals with Blood Type A, incorporating herbal teas and infusions into their daily routine can provide numerous health benefits. These natural remedies support digestion, boost immunity, and promote relaxation. Selecting the right herbal teas that align with the Blood Type A dietary recommendations can enhance overall well-being.

Chamomile tea is highly beneficial for Blood Type A individuals. It has soothing properties that help reduce stress and promote restful sleep. Chamomile also aids in digestion and can alleviate stomach discomfort. Drinking a cup of chamomile tea in the evening can help calm the mind and prepare the body for a good night's sleep.

Green tea is another excellent choice. It is rich in antioxidants, which support the immune system and protect against cellular damage. Green tea also has anti-inflammatory properties and can aid in weight management by boosting metabolism. Drinking green tea regularly can enhance mental clarity and provide sustained energy throughout the day.

Ginger tea is particularly effective for digestive health. It helps stimulate digestion, reduce nausea, and alleviate bloating. Ginger's anti-inflammatory properties also support joint health and can relieve muscle soreness. A cup of ginger tea after meals can aid in digestion and provide relief from digestive discomfort.

Licorice root tea is beneficial for its soothing and anti-inflammatory properties. It can help alleviate symptoms of digestive disorders such as acid reflux and gastritis. Licorice root also supports adrenal health, helping the body cope with stress. Drinking licorice root tea can provide a calming effect and support overall digestive health.

Peppermint tea is excellent for relieving digestive issues such as bloating, gas, and indigestion. It has a cooling effect that can soothe the stomach and relax the digestive tract muscles. Peppermint tea also has a refreshing flavor and can help alleviate headaches and improve mental focus.

Rooibos tea, also known as red bush tea, is rich in antioxidants and free from caffeine. It supports cardiovascular health, aids in digestion, and promotes relaxation. Rooibos tea is also known for its anti-inflammatory properties, making it an excellent choice for Blood Type A individuals looking to reduce inflammation and support overall health.

Dandelion root tea is a powerful detoxifier. It supports liver health by promoting bile production and aiding in the elimination of toxins from the body. Dandelion root also has diuretic properties, helping to reduce water retention and support kidney function. Drinking dandelion root tea regularly can enhance liver function and promote detoxification.

Nettle tea is highly nutritious and rich in vitamins and minerals such as iron, calcium, and magnesium. It supports overall health by boosting the immune system, reducing inflammation, and improving energy levels. Nettle tea can also help alleviate allergy symptoms and support skin health.

Hibiscus tea is known for its vibrant color and tangy flavor. It is rich in antioxidants and vitamin C, which support the immune system and promote skin health. Hibiscus tea also has antihypertensive properties, helping to lower blood pressure and support cardiovascular health. Drinking hibiscus tea can provide a refreshing and health-boosting beverage option.

Lemon balm tea is excellent for reducing stress and promoting relaxation. It has mild sedative properties that can help improve sleep quality and reduce anxiety. Lemon balm tea also supports digestive health by alleviating symptoms of indigestion and bloating. Drinking lemon balm tea can help create a sense of calm and well-being.

Valerian root tea is a natural remedy for promoting relaxation and improving sleep. It has sedative properties that can help reduce anxiety and improve sleep quality. Valerian root tea is especially beneficial for individuals with Blood Type A who may experience stress and tension. Drinking valerian root tea in the evening can support restful sleep and relaxation.

Milk thistle tea is known for its liver-protective properties. It helps detoxify the liver and support its function. Milk thistle tea also has anti-inflammatory properties and can aid in digestion. Drinking milk thistle tea regularly can support liver health and enhance the body's natural detoxification processes.

Fennel tea is beneficial for digestive health. It helps reduce bloating, gas, and indigestion. Fennel tea also has anti-inflammatory properties and can support respiratory health by alleviating symptoms of bronchitis and asthma. Drinking fennel tea after meals can aid in digestion and provide relief from digestive discomfort.

Holy basil tea, also known as tulsi tea, is an adaptogen that helps the body cope with stress. It supports immune function, reduces inflammation, and promotes mental clarity. Holy basil tea can also help balance blood sugar levels and support cardiovascular health. Drinking holy basil tea regularly can enhance overall well-being and resilience to stress.

By incorporating these herbal teas and infusions into your diet, you can support various aspects of your health and well-being. Each tea offers unique benefits that align with the needs of Blood Type A individuals, helping to create a balanced and health-promoting daily routine.

# Exercise Recommendations

## Best Types of Exercise for Blood Type A

For individuals with Blood Type A, incorporating the right types of exercise into their routine is essential for maintaining optimal health and well-being. Blood Type A individuals tend to thrive on exercises that promote relaxation, reduce stress, and enhance overall physical and mental health. Here are the best types of exercises for Blood Type A:

Yoga is an excellent form of exercise for Blood Type A individuals. It promotes relaxation, reduces stress, and improves flexibility and strength. Practicing yoga regularly can help balance the mind and body, making it an ideal choice for maintaining overall health. Incorporating yoga sessions into your weekly routine can enhance your mental clarity and reduce stress levels, which is particularly beneficial for Blood Type A individuals who may be prone to higher stress levels.

Tai Chi is another highly recommended exercise for Blood Type A. This ancient Chinese martial art focuses on slow, controlled movements and deep breathing techniques. Tai Chi helps improve balance, flexibility, and mental focus. It is a low-impact exercise that is gentle on the joints, making it suitable for all fitness levels. Regular practice of Tai Chi can help reduce stress, improve circulation, and promote a sense of calm and well-being.

Pilates is beneficial for Blood Type A individuals as it focuses on core strength, flexibility, and overall body awareness. Pilates exercises emphasize controlled movements and proper breathing, which can help reduce stress and improve posture. Incorporating Pilates into your exercise routine can enhance your core stability, increase muscle tone, and improve overall physical fitness.

Walking is a simple yet effective exercise for Blood Type A individuals. It is a low-impact activity that can be easily incorporated into daily routines. Walking helps improve cardiovascular health, boosts mood, and reduces stress. Aim for at least 30 minutes of brisk walking each day to enjoy the physical and mental health benefits. Walking in nature or green spaces can further enhance the stress-reducing benefits of this activity.

Swimming is an excellent full-body workout for Blood Type A individuals. It is a low-impact exercise that improves cardiovascular fitness, builds muscle strength, and enhances flexibility. Swimming can also help reduce stress and promote relaxation. Incorporating regular swimming sessions into your exercise routine can improve overall physical fitness and mental well-being.

Cycling is another great option for Blood Type A individuals. It is a low-impact cardiovascular exercise that can help improve heart health, build muscle strength, and boost endurance. Cycling can be done outdoors or indoors on a stationary bike. Regular cycling can help reduce stress levels and improve overall physical fitness.

Stretching exercises are essential for Blood Type A individuals to maintain flexibility and reduce muscle tension. Incorporating a regular stretching routine can help improve joint range of motion, prevent injuries, and promote relaxation. Stretching can be done as a standalone activity or as part of a warm-up or cool-down routine for other exercises.

Moderate aerobic exercises, such as dancing, are also beneficial for Blood Type A individuals. These activities help improve cardiovascular health, boost mood, and reduce stress. Participating in dance classes or simply dancing at home can be a fun and effective way to stay active and maintain overall health.

Strength training with light weights is recommended for Blood Type A individuals to build muscle strength and improve bone density. Using light weights and focusing on controlled movements can help avoid injury and promote overall physical fitness. Incorporating strength training exercises into your routine two to three times a week can enhance muscle tone and support a healthy metabolism.

Mind-body exercises, such as meditation, are crucial for Blood Type A individuals. Regular meditation practice can help reduce stress, improve mental clarity, and promote a sense of inner peace. Incorporating meditation into your daily routine can enhance overall well-being and complement other forms of physical exercise.

By focusing on these types of exercises, Blood Type A individuals can maintain a balanced and healthy lifestyle. These exercises not only support physical health but also promote mental and emotional well-being, which is essential for overall health and longevity.

# Creating an Exercise Routine

Creating an exercise routine for individuals with Blood Type A involves focusing on activities that promote relaxation, reduce stress, and enhance overall well-being. Blood Type A individuals often thrive with a more gentle and meditative approach to exercise. This is because they tend to have higher levels of the stress hormone cortisol, making it essential to engage in activities that lower stress and promote a calm state of mind.

Yoga is highly recommended for Blood Type A individuals as it combines physical postures, breathing exercises, and meditation. It helps reduce stress, improve flexibility, and increase strength. Practicing yoga regularly can enhance mental clarity, boost immune function, and improve digestion. Aim to incorporate yoga sessions into your routine at least three to four times a week. Start with beginner-friendly poses and gradually move to more advanced postures as your flexibility and strength improve.

Tai Chi is another excellent exercise option. This ancient Chinese practice focuses on slow, deliberate movements, deep breathing, and meditation. Tai Chi helps balance the mind and body, reduce stress, and improve overall health. Regular practice can enhance coordination, balance, and muscle strength. For optimal benefits, practice Tai Chi for 30 to 60 minutes, three to five times a week.

Pilates offers a low-impact workout that strengthens the core, improves posture, and enhances flexibility. It focuses on controlled movements and breathing, making it ideal for Blood Type A individuals. Incorporating Pilates into your routine can help alleviate stress, support joint health, and increase overall body awareness. Aim to practice Pilates two to three times a week, either through classes or guided videos.

Walking is a simple yet effective exercise that provides numerous health benefits. It is an excellent way to reduce stress, improve cardiovascular health, and maintain a healthy weight. Walking outdoors also allows you to connect with nature, further promoting relaxation and mental well-being. Aim for 30 to 45 minutes of brisk walking five to six times a week. Consider incorporating walking into your daily routine, such as walking to work or taking a stroll after meals.

Swimming is a full-body workout that is gentle on the joints and ideal for Blood Type A individuals. It helps improve cardiovascular fitness, build muscle strength, and enhance flexibility. Swimming can also be a meditative activity, promoting relaxation and reducing stress. Try to swim for 30 to 60 minutes, three to four times a week, to reap the maximum benefits.

Cycling, whether outdoors or on a stationary bike, provides a low-impact cardiovascular workout that is suitable for Blood Type A individuals. It helps improve heart health, build leg strength, and boost endurance. Cycling can be a relaxing activity, especially when done in scenic areas. Aim for 30 to 45 minutes of cycling three to four times a week.

Strength training, using light weights or resistance bands, can help Blood Type A individuals build muscle strength and improve bone density without putting excessive stress on the body. Focus on exercises that target major muscle groups, such as squats, lunges, and push-ups. Perform strength training sessions two to three times a week, with a focus on proper form and controlled movements.

Incorporating mindfulness practices, such as meditation and deep breathing exercises, into your exercise routine can further enhance the stress-reducing benefits. Spend 10 to 15 minutes each day practicing mindfulness to calm the mind, improve concentration, and promote a sense of inner peace. These practices can be done before or after your physical exercise sessions to enhance overall well-being.

Blood Type A individuals should avoid high-intensity workouts that can elevate cortisol levels and increase stress. Instead, focus on exercises that promote relaxation, improve flexibility, and support cardiovascular health. Consistency is key, so aim to create a balanced routine that includes a variety of activities to keep both your body and mind engaged.

By following these exercise recommendations and incorporating them into your daily routine, Blood Type A individuals can achieve better physical and mental health, reduce stress, and enhance overall quality of life.

# Mind Body Practices: Yoga and Meditation

For individuals with Blood Type A, engaging in mind-body practices such as yoga and meditation is particularly beneficial. These practices align well with the dietary guidelines in the Blood Type A Food List, promoting a holistic approach to health and wellness. Yoga and meditation help manage stress, improve mental clarity, and enhance physical well-being, making them ideal exercise recommendations for Blood Type A individuals.

Yoga is a practice that combines physical postures, breathing exercises, and meditation. It is known for its ability to reduce stress, improve flexibility, and enhance overall physical health. For Blood Type A individuals, yoga offers a gentle yet effective way to maintain fitness without overexertion. The focus on breath control and mindful movement helps in managing the stress levels that Blood Type A individuals are particularly sensitive to. Regular yoga practice can improve circulation, strengthen muscles, and support a healthy immune system.

There are various styles of yoga to choose from, each catering to different fitness levels and preferences. Hatha yoga, for instance, is a slower-paced practice that emphasizes gentle stretching and breath work, making it ideal for beginners and those seeking a calming exercise routine. Vinyasa yoga, on the other hand, involves a more dynamic flow of movements synchronized with breath, providing a moderate cardiovascular workout. Restorative yoga focuses on deep relaxation and the use of props to support the body, which can be particularly beneficial for stress relief and recovery.

Meditation complements yoga by further promoting mental clarity and emotional stability. Blood Type A individuals often benefit from meditation due to their higher susceptibility to stress and anxiety. Meditation practices involve focusing the mind and eliminating distractions to achieve a state of relaxation and heightened awareness. This practice can help reduce cortisol levels, improve concentration, and enhance emotional resilience.

There are several forms of meditation that can be easily incorporated into daily routines. Mindfulness meditation involves paying attention to the present moment without judgment. This practice helps Blood Type A individuals develop a greater awareness of their thoughts and feelings, leading to better stress management and emotional regulation. Guided meditation, where an instructor or recording leads the participant through a series of visualizations and breathing exercises, can be particularly helpful for beginners or those looking for structure in their practice.

Another beneficial form of meditation is transcendental meditation, which involves the use of a mantra to focus the mind and achieve a deep state of rest and relaxation. This technique has been shown to reduce stress and promote overall well-being, making it an excellent choice for Blood Type A individuals. Practicing meditation regularly can improve sleep quality, enhance cognitive function, and support emotional balance.

Combining yoga and meditation provides a comprehensive approach to fitness and wellness for Blood Type A individuals. Practicing yoga several times a week can help maintain physical health, while daily meditation sessions support mental and emotional well-being. Together, these practices create a balanced routine that addresses the unique needs of Blood Type A individuals, promoting a harmonious mind-body connection.

Incorporating these mind-body practices into a weekly routine is straightforward. Start with a short, manageable yoga session, such as a 20-minute Hatha yoga practice, and gradually increase the duration and intensity as comfort and fitness levels improve. Follow the yoga session with a 10-minute mindfulness meditation to enhance relaxation and mental clarity. Over time, extend meditation sessions to 20 or 30 minutes for deeper benefits.

By integrating yoga and meditation into their lifestyle, Blood Type A individuals can significantly enhance their overall health. These practices help manage stress, improve physical fitness, and promote a sense of inner peace and balance. Coupled with the dietary recommendations in the Blood Type A Food List, yoga and meditation offer a holistic approach to achieving optimal health and well-being.

# Stress Management

## Techniques for Reducing Stress

Stress management is crucial for individuals with Blood Type A, as they tend to have a more sensitive immune system and higher stress levels. Implementing effective stress-reduction techniques can help maintain overall health and well-being. Here are several techniques specifically beneficial for those following the Blood Type A food list.

Mindfulness meditation involves focusing on the present moment and accepting it without judgment. This practice can significantly reduce stress by promoting relaxation and mental clarity. Individuals with Blood Type A can benefit from setting aside 10-20 minutes daily to practice mindfulness meditation in a quiet space, focusing on their breath and allowing thoughts to pass without attachment.

Yoga combines physical postures, breathing exercises, and meditation to enhance physical and mental well-being. For Blood Type A individuals, gentle yoga practices such as Hatha or Restorative Yoga are particularly beneficial. These styles focus on slow movements and deep relaxation, helping to reduce stress and improve flexibility. Practicing yoga for 30-60 minutes a few times a week can significantly lower stress levels.

Deep breathing exercises can help activate the body's relaxation response, reducing stress and anxiety. Techniques such as diaphragmatic breathing, where one breathes deeply into the abdomen, can be practiced anywhere and anytime. Blood Type A individuals can incorporate deep breathing exercises into their daily routine, spending a few minutes focusing on slow, deep breaths to calm the nervous system.

Progressive muscle relaxation involves tensing and then slowly relaxing each muscle group in the body. This technique can help reduce physical tension and promote a state of relaxation. Blood Type A individuals can practice progressive muscle relaxation by lying down in a comfortable position, starting with the muscles in their toes, and working up to their head, tensing and relaxing each muscle group for a few seconds.

Tai Chi is a form of martial arts that focuses on slow, deliberate movements and deep breathing. This practice can improve balance, flexibility, and mental focus while reducing stress. Blood Type A individuals can benefit from practicing Tai Chi regularly, either by joining a class or following along with instructional videos, dedicating 20-30 minutes to practice a few times a week.

Guided imagery involves visualizing calming and peaceful images to reduce stress. This technique can help Blood Type A individuals escape from daily stressors and promote a sense of relaxation. They can practice guided imagery by listening to recordings or following scripts that guide them through peaceful scenes, such as walking through a forest or lying on a beach, focusing on the sensory details of these environments.

Adequate sleep is essential for stress management, as lack of sleep can exacerbate stress levels. Blood Type A individuals should aim for 7-9 hours of quality sleep each night. Establishing a regular sleep schedule, creating a relaxing bedtime routine, and ensuring a comfortable sleep environment can help improve sleep quality and reduce stress.

Regular physical activity can help reduce stress by releasing endorphins and promoting overall well-being. Blood Type A individuals should engage in moderate-intensity exercises such as walking, cycling, or swimming for at least 30 minutes most days of the week. These activities can help reduce stress hormones and improve mood.

Maintaining a healthy diet is also crucial for managing stress. Blood Type A individuals should follow the recommended dietary guidelines, focusing on plant-based proteins, vegetables, and fruits, while avoiding foods that can cause inflammation and stress. Eating balanced meals at regular intervals can help stabilize blood sugar levels and reduce stress.

Social support is vital for stress management. Blood Type A individuals should nurture relationships with family, friends, and support groups. Engaging in social activities, sharing feelings, and seeking support during stressful times can provide emotional relief and reduce feelings of isolation.

By incorporating these stress-reduction techniques into their daily routine, individuals with Blood Type A can effectively manage stress, improve their overall health, and enhance their quality of life.

# The Importance of Relaxation

Relaxation is crucial for individuals with Blood Type A, as their sensitive and often stress-prone nature can lead to various health issues if not properly managed. Incorporating effective relaxation techniques into daily life can significantly enhance overall well-being and support the positive effects of the Blood Type A diet.

One of the key reasons relaxation is essential for Blood Type A individuals is the impact of stress on their digestive system. Chronic stress can disrupt digestion, leading to issues such as bloating, gas, and stomach pain. By practicing relaxation techniques, the body can enter a state of rest and digest, which optimizes digestive function and enhances nutrient absorption from the foods consumed.

Moreover, stress negatively affects the immune system, making Blood Type A individuals more susceptible to illnesses. Relaxation helps to reduce the production of stress hormones like cortisol, which can suppress immune function. Regular relaxation practices can boost the immune system, allowing the body to better defend itself against infections and diseases.

Mental health is another area where relaxation plays a significant role. Blood Type A individuals often have a predisposition to anxiety and heightened emotional responses. Engaging in relaxation activities such as deep breathing exercises, meditation, and yoga can help calm the mind, reduce anxiety levels, and promote emotional stability. This mental clarity and peace contribute to overall well-being and better decision-making regarding diet and lifestyle choices.

Physical health is directly impacted by stress, with prolonged stress contributing to increased blood pressure, heart disease, and other chronic conditions. For Blood Type A individuals, who may already be at a higher risk for cardiovascular issues, relaxation is vital for maintaining heart health. Techniques like progressive muscle relaxation, tai chi, and regular physical activity tailored to their needs can lower blood pressure, improve circulation, and promote cardiovascular health.

Incorporating relaxation into daily routines can also enhance sleep quality. Stress often leads to sleep disturbances, which can further exacerbate health issues. Blood Type A individuals benefit from relaxation techniques such as a consistent bedtime routine, limiting screen time before bed, and practicing mindfulness or gentle stretching. Improved sleep quality supports overall health, aiding in recovery, reducing inflammation, and enhancing cognitive function.

Additionally, relaxation can improve relationships and social interactions. Stress often strains relationships and reduces the ability to connect with others. By managing stress through relaxation, Blood Type A individuals can foster better communication, empathy, and social bonds. This social support network is essential for emotional health and can provide motivation and encouragement in adhering to a healthy lifestyle.

Finally, incorporating relaxation techniques into a holistic approach to health aligns with the principles of the Blood Type A diet. Just as certain foods are chosen to support optimal health, specific relaxation practices are selected to address the unique needs of Blood Type A individuals. This comprehensive approach ensures that both diet and lifestyle work synergistically to promote overall wellness.

In summary, the importance of relaxation for Blood Type A individuals cannot be overstated. It supports digestive health, boosts the immune system, improves mental and physical well-being, enhances sleep quality, and fosters better relationships. By prioritizing relaxation alongside dietary choices, Blood Type A individuals can achieve a balanced and healthy lifestyle.

# Breathing Exercises and Meditation

For individuals with Blood Type A, managing stress is crucial for overall health and well-being. Incorporating breathing exercises and meditation into your daily routine can significantly reduce stress levels, promote relaxation, and enhance mental clarity. These practices help calm the nervous system, regulate the body's response to stress, and improve overall emotional balance.

Breathing exercises are a simple yet effective way to manage stress. Deep breathing, also known as diaphragmatic breathing or abdominal breathing, involves taking slow, deep breaths that fill the lungs completely. This type of breathing stimulates the parasympathetic nervous system, which is responsible for the body's rest-and-digest response. To practice deep breathing, sit or lie down in a comfortable position, place one hand on your chest and the other on your abdomen, inhale deeply through your nose, allowing your abdomen to rise, and then exhale slowly through your mouth, allowing your abdomen to fall. Repeat this process for several minutes, focusing on the sensation of the breath entering and leaving your body.

Alternate nostril breathing, or Nadi Shodhana, is another beneficial technique. This practice balances the left and right hemispheres of the brain, promoting mental clarity and emotional stability. To perform alternate nostril breathing, sit in a comfortable position, use your right thumb to close your right nostril, inhale deeply through your left nostril, close your left nostril with your right ring finger, release your right nostril, and exhale through your right nostril. Then, inhale through your right nostril, close it with your right thumb, release your left nostril, and exhale through your left nostril. Continue this pattern for several minutes.

Box breathing, also known as four-square breathing, is a technique used to calm the mind and reduce stress. This method involves inhaling for a count of four, holding the breath for a count of four, exhaling for a count of four, and holding the breath again for a count of four. This rhythmic breathing pattern can help regulate the body's stress response and promote a sense of calm. To practice box breathing, sit comfortably, inhale through your nose for a count of four, hold your breath for a count of four, exhale through your mouth for a count of four, and hold your breath again for a count of four. Repeat this cycle several times, focusing on the steady rhythm of your breath.

Meditation is another powerful tool for stress management. Mindfulness meditation involves paying attention to the present moment without judgment. This practice can help reduce anxiety, improve concentration, and enhance emotional regulation. To practice mindfulness meditation, find a quiet place to sit or lie down, close your eyes, and bring your attention to your breath. Notice the sensation of the breath as it enters and leaves your nostrils or the rise and fall of your abdomen. Whenever your mind wanders, gently bring your focus back to your breath. Practice this for several minutes each day, gradually increasing the duration as you become more comfortable with the practice.

Guided meditation involves listening to a recording or a guide who leads you through a series of visualizations or relaxation techniques. This type of meditation can be especially helpful for beginners or those who find it difficult to focus on their own. There are many resources available online, including apps and videos, that offer guided meditations tailored to various needs and preferences. To practice guided meditation, find a comfortable position, put on headphones if desired, and follow the instructions provided by the guide. Allow yourself to fully immerse in the experience and let go of any tension or stress.

Loving-kindness meditation, also known as Metta meditation, involves focusing on developing feelings of compassion and love towards oneself and others. This practice can enhance emotional well-being and foster a sense of connectedness. To practice loving-kindness meditation, sit comfortably, close your eyes, and bring to mind someone you care about. Silently repeat phrases such as "May you be happy, may you be healthy, may you be safe, may you live with ease." After a few minutes, extend these wishes to yourself and then to others, including those you may have difficulties with. Practice this for several minutes, cultivating feelings of love and compassion.

Incorporating these breathing exercises and meditation practices into your daily routine can help Blood Type A individuals effectively manage stress, promote relaxation, and enhance overall health. By dedicating time each day to these practices, you can create a sense of inner peace and resilience that supports your well-being.

# 21 Days Meal Plan

**Day 1**

- **Breakfast:** Green smoothie with spinach, banana, almond milk, and chia seeds
- **Lunch:** Quinoa salad with mixed greens, cherry tomatoes, cucumbers, and tofu
- **Dinner:** Grilled salmon with steamed broccoli and sweet potato
- **Snacks:** Apple slices with almond butter

**Day 2**

- **Breakfast:** Overnight oats with blueberries, flaxseeds, and almond milk
- **Lunch:** Lentil soup with carrots, celery, and onions
- **Dinner:** Stir-fried vegetables with tempeh and brown rice
- **Snacks:** Carrot sticks with hummus

**Day 3**

- **Breakfast:** Greek yogurt with honey, walnuts, and strawberries
- **Lunch:** Mixed bean salad with chickpeas, black beans, corn, and avocado
- **Dinner:** Baked tofu with roasted Brussels sprouts and quinoa

- **Snacks:** Mixed berries

**Day 4**

- **Breakfast:** Smoothie bowl with acai, banana, almond milk, and granola
- **Lunch:** Spinach and kale salad with roasted butternut squash and pumpkin seeds
- **Dinner:** Grilled mackerel with asparagus and brown rice
- **Snacks:** Rice cakes with almond butter

**Day 5**

- **Breakfast:** Avocado toast on whole grain bread with a side of fresh fruit
- **Lunch:** Chickpea and vegetable stir-fry with brown rice
- **Dinner:** Baked cod with green beans and mashed sweet potatoes
- **Snacks:** Sliced cucumbers with hummus

**Day 6**

- **Breakfast:** Chia pudding with almond milk, vanilla extract, and fresh berries
- **Lunch:** Lentil and quinoa bowl with roasted vegetables
- **Dinner:** Stir-fried tofu with bell peppers and broccoli, served with brown rice
- **Snacks:** Apple slices with tahini

**Day 7**

- **Breakfast:** Smoothie with kale, mango, banana, and hemp seeds
- **Lunch:** Mediterranean quinoa salad with cucumbers, tomatoes, olives, and feta cheese
- **Dinner:** Baked salmon with steamed spinach and quinoa
- **Snacks:** Almonds and dried apricots

**Day 8**

- **Breakfast:** Oatmeal with cinnamon, flaxseeds, and sliced banana
- **Lunch:** Tofu and vegetable wrap with hummus
- **Dinner:** Grilled shrimp with asparagus and wild rice
- **Snacks:** Bell pepper slices with guacamole

**Day 9**

- **Breakfast:** Green smoothie with spinach, pineapple, coconut water, and chia seeds
- **Lunch:** Lentil and vegetable stew with a side of whole grain bread
- **Dinner:** Baked trout with roasted sweet potatoes and green beans
- **Snacks:** Mixed nuts

**Day 10**

- **Breakfast:** Smoothie bowl with acai, banana, almond milk, and granola
- **Lunch:** Spinach salad with roasted beets, walnuts, and goat cheese
- **Dinner:** Grilled tofu with stir-fried vegetables and brown rice
- **Snacks:** Celery sticks with almond butter

**Day 11**

- **Breakfast:** Greek yogurt with honey, walnuts, and strawberries
- **Lunch:** Chickpea and avocado salad with mixed greens
- **Dinner:** Baked mackerel with steamed broccoli and quinoa
- **Snacks:** Apple slices with tahini

**Day 12**

- **Breakfast:** Avocado toast on whole grain bread with a side of fresh fruit
- **Lunch:** Quinoa and vegetable bowl with roasted chickpeas
- **Dinner:** Grilled salmon with green beans and wild rice
- **Snacks:** Sliced cucumbers with hummus

**Day 13**

- **Breakfast:** Chia pudding with almond milk, vanilla extract, and fresh berries

- **Lunch:** Lentil soup with carrots, celery, and onions
- **Dinner:** Baked tofu with roasted Brussels sprouts and quinoa
- **Snacks:** Rice cakes with almond butter

## Day 14

- **Breakfast:** Smoothie with kale, mango, banana, and hemp seeds
- **Lunch:** Mixed bean salad with chickpeas, black beans, corn, and avocado
- **Dinner:** Grilled mackerel with asparagus and brown rice
- **Snacks:** Almonds and dried apricots

## Day 15

- **Breakfast:** Oatmeal with cinnamon, flaxseeds, and sliced banana
- **Lunch:** Tofu and vegetable wrap with hummus
- **Dinner:** Baked cod with green beans and mashed sweet potatoes
- **Snacks:** Carrot sticks with hummus

## Day 16

- **Breakfast:** Green smoothie with spinach, pineapple, coconut water, and chia seeds
- **Lunch:** Spinach and kale salad with roasted butternut squash and pumpkin seeds

- **Dinner:** Grilled shrimp with asparagus and wild rice
- **Snacks:** Mixed nuts

**Day 17**

- **Breakfast:** Smoothie bowl with acai, banana, almond milk, and granola
- **Lunch:** Lentil and quinoa bowl with roasted vegetables
- **Dinner:** Stir-fried tofu with bell peppers and broccoli, served with brown rice
- **Snacks:** Celery sticks with almond butter

**Day 18**

- **Breakfast:** Greek yogurt with honey, walnuts, and strawberries
- **Lunch:** Mediterranean quinoa salad with cucumbers, tomatoes, olives, and feta cheese
- **Dinner:** Baked trout with roasted sweet potatoes and green beans
- **Snacks:** Sliced cucumbers with hummus

**Day 19**

- **Breakfast:** Avocado toast on whole grain bread with a side of fresh fruit
- **Lunch:** Chickpea and vegetable stir-fry with brown rice
- **Dinner:** Grilled tofu with steamed spinach and quinoa

- **Snacks:** Apple slices with tahini

**Day 20**

- **Breakfast:** Chia pudding with almond milk, vanilla extract, and fresh berries
- **Lunch:** Spinach salad with roasted beets, walnuts, and goat cheese
- **Dinner:** Baked salmon with green beans and wild rice
- **Snacks:** Mixed nuts

**Day 21**

- **Breakfast:** Smoothie with kale, mango, banana, and hemp seeds
- **Lunch:** Quinoa salad with mixed greens, cherry tomatoes, cucumbers, and tofu
- **Dinner:** Grilled mackerel with asparagus and brown rice
- **Snacks:** Bell pepper slices with guacamole

# Cooking Techniques

## Best Cooking Methods for Blood Type A

For individuals with Blood Type A, choosing the right cooking methods is essential to preserve the nutritional value of foods and support overall health. Certain techniques are more beneficial as they enhance the digestibility of food, retain essential nutrients, and reduce the formation of harmful compounds.

Steaming is one of the best cooking methods for Blood Type A individuals. It helps retain the maximum amount of nutrients in vegetables and prevents the loss of water-soluble vitamins. Steaming vegetables, fish, and poultry ensures that the food remains tender and easy to digest, which is ideal for the sensitive digestive system of Blood Type A individuals. This method also reduces the need for added fats and oils, promoting a healthier diet.

Sautéing is another effective cooking technique that can be beneficial. Using a small amount of healthy oil, such as olive oil or flaxseed oil, can enhance the flavor of vegetables, tofu, and lean proteins without overwhelming the dish with unhealthy fats. It is important to use low to medium heat to avoid burning the oil and forming harmful compounds. Sautéing can quickly cook food, preserving its texture and nutritional content.

Baking is a versatile and healthy cooking method. Baking fish, poultry, and vegetables at moderate temperatures can help retain their natural flavors and nutrients. Using herbs and spices instead of excessive salt and unhealthy fats can enhance the taste while keeping the meal nutritious. Baking allows for even cooking and can be a convenient way to prepare meals in advance.

Poaching is particularly suitable for cooking delicate proteins like fish and eggs. Poaching in water or broth at a low temperature helps preserve the texture and moisture of the food. This gentle cooking method minimizes the formation of harmful compounds and is easy on the digestive system. It is an excellent way to prepare light and healthy dishes.

Grilling, when done properly, can be a healthy cooking method. It is important to grill at lower temperatures to avoid charring, which can produce harmful substances. Marinating proteins like chicken or fish in lemon juice, herbs, and olive oil before grilling can add flavor and reduce the formation of potentially harmful compounds. Using a grill pan or an indoor grill can help control the cooking temperature and reduce exposure to open flames.

Slow cooking is ideal for preparing stews, soups, and casseroles. This method allows ingredients to cook slowly at a low temperature, preserving their nutrients and enhancing flavors. Slow cooking is especially useful for legumes and tougher cuts of meat, making them tender and easy to digest. It is also a convenient way to prepare large batches of food.

Stir-frying can be a quick and healthy cooking method if done correctly. Using a small amount of healthy oil and high heat, stir-frying can cook vegetables and lean proteins quickly, preserving their nutrients and crisp texture. It is important to keep the cooking time short to avoid overcooking and nutrient loss. Adding a variety of colorful vegetables can make the dish more nutritious and appealing.

Blanching is useful for preparing vegetables while retaining their bright color and nutrients. Briefly boiling vegetables and then plunging them into ice water stops the cooking process and locks in nutrients. Blanching can be a great way to prepare vegetables for salads, stir-fries, or as a healthy snack.

Using a pressure cooker can significantly reduce cooking times while preserving nutrients. This method is particularly effective for cooking legumes, grains, and tougher cuts of meat. Pressure cooking helps retain vitamins and minerals that might be lost during longer cooking processes and ensures that food is tender and easy to digest.

Fermenting is a valuable technique for Blood Type A individuals. Fermented foods like sauerkraut, kimchi, and miso are rich in probiotics, which support gut health and digestion. Fermentation enhances the nutritional profile of foods and makes them easier to digest, which is beneficial for the sensitive digestive system of Blood Type A individuals.

By focusing on these cooking methods, Blood Type A individuals can maximize the nutritional value of their meals, support their digestive health, and enjoy a varied and flavorful diet. These techniques help retain essential nutrients, reduce the formation of harmful compounds, and enhance the overall quality of the diet.

# Tips for Healthy Cooking

For individuals with Blood Type A, using healthy cooking techniques is essential to maximize the nutritional benefits of your food and maintain overall well-being. Adopting specific methods can enhance the digestibility and nutrient retention of your meals, which is particularly important for those following the Blood Type A Food List. Here are some tips for healthy cooking tailored to Blood Type A dietary guidelines.

Opt for steaming vegetables as this method preserves essential vitamins and minerals while making the vegetables easier to digest. Steaming broccoli, spinach, and carrots ensures that you get the maximum health benefits without the loss of nutrients that can occur with boiling or frying.

Choose baking or roasting as these methods use dry heat, which can help retain the flavor and nutrients of your food. For example, baking tofu with a light marinade or roasting sweet potatoes with a sprinkle of olive oil and herbs can create delicious, nutrient-dense dishes without the need for unhealthy fats.

Incorporate sautéing with healthy oils such as olive oil or flaxseed oil. These oils are beneficial for Blood Type A individuals and can add flavor and healthy fats to your meals. When sautéing vegetables or lean proteins like chicken or fish, use moderate heat to prevent the breakdown of these oils into harmful compounds.

Experiment with slow cooking or using a pressure cooker to prepare legumes and grains. Slow cooking black beans or lentils ensures they are thoroughly cooked and easier to digest, which is crucial for Blood Type A individuals who may have sensitive digestive systems. Pressure cooking grains like quinoa can also reduce cooking time while preserving nutrients.

Make use of blending for soups and smoothies. Blending helps break down fibers, making them easier to digest and allowing for better absorption of nutrients. For example, a smoothie with spinach, berries, and chia seeds provides a nutrient-rich, easily digestible meal. Similarly, blended vegetable soups can be both comforting and nutritious.

Ferment foods to enhance their probiotic content. Fermented foods like miso, tempeh, and sauerkraut are excellent for Blood Type A individuals as they support gut health. Incorporate these foods into your diet by adding miso to soups, using tempeh in stir-fries, or serving sauerkraut as a side dish.

Avoid deep frying as it involves high temperatures and unhealthy fats that can cause inflammation and digestive issues for Blood Type A individuals. Instead, use air frying as a healthier alternative. Air frying can create a crispy texture without the excessive use of oil, making it suitable for preparing vegetables, tofu, and even lean meats.

Practice marinating to enhance flavor and tenderize proteins. Marinating chicken or fish in a mixture of olive oil, lemon juice, and herbs can add flavor without the need for excessive salt or unhealthy additives. Marinating also helps break down proteins, making them easier to digest for Blood Type A individuals.

Incorporate poaching for delicate proteins such as fish and eggs. Poaching involves cooking food in simmering water or broth, which helps retain moisture and nutrients. Poached salmon or eggs can be a gentle, nutritious option for Blood Type A individuals.

Use herbs and spices generously to add flavor and health benefits to your dishes. Herbs like garlic, ginger, turmeric, and parsley not only enhance the taste but also provide anti-inflammatory and antioxidant properties. These herbs and spices can be particularly beneficial for Blood Type A individuals.

Ensure proper portion control to maintain a balanced diet. For Blood Type A individuals, it is important to focus on portion sizes to avoid overeating and ensure a variety of nutrients. Using smaller plates and measuring portions can help achieve this balance.

Emphasize hydration by incorporating water-rich foods and soups into your meals. Foods like cucumbers, leafy greens, and broth-based soups can contribute to overall hydration, which is vital for digestive health and overall well-being.

By adopting these healthy cooking techniques, Blood Type A individuals can create delicious, nutrient-dense meals that support their unique dietary needs. These methods not only enhance the flavor and texture of foods but also ensure the preservation and optimal absorption of essential nutrients.

# Adapting Recipes to Fit the Diet

Adapting recipes to fit the Blood Type A diet involves making thoughtful substitutions and adjustments to ensure meals are both compliant with dietary guidelines and delicious. The focus is on using plant-based proteins, avoiding harmful fats, and incorporating beneficial foods that support overall health and well-being. Here are some detailed strategies and techniques to help adapt recipes for Blood Type A:

Substitute animal proteins with plant-based options. Instead of using red meat or pork, opt for tofu, tempeh, lentils, or beans. These alternatives are rich in protein and easier to digest for Blood Type A individuals. For example, in a stir-fry recipe, replace chicken with tofu cubes or tempeh slices. Marinate the tofu or tempeh in soy sauce, ginger, and garlic to enhance flavor before cooking.

Replace dairy products with plant-based alternatives. Blood Type A individuals often have difficulty digesting dairy, so substitute cow's milk with almond milk, soy milk, or oat milk. Use these alternatives in baking, smoothies, or cereal. For creamy sauces, blend soaked cashews with water to create a rich, dairy-free cream. This can be used in recipes like creamy pasta sauces or soups.

Use healthy oils and fats. Avoid oils high in omega-6 fatty acids and trans fats, such as corn oil, soybean oil, and margarine. Instead, use olive oil, flaxseed oil, or avocado oil for cooking and salad dressings. These oils are beneficial for Blood Type A and provide essential fatty acids without promoting inflammation. For example, sauté vegetables in olive oil or drizzle flaxseed oil over salads.

Incorporate beneficial grains. Replace refined grains and wheat products with whole grains like quinoa, brown rice, and amaranth. These grains are more suitable for Blood Type A and provide essential nutrients and fiber. Use quinoa as a base for salads, brown rice in stir-fries, and amaranth in porridge or as a side dish.

Enhance flavor with herbs and spices. Blood Type A individuals can benefit from using a variety of herbs and spices that aid digestion and boost immunity. Incorporate garlic, ginger, turmeric, and parsley into your recipes. For instance, add minced garlic and grated ginger to soups, stews, and marinades. Use turmeric in curries and sprinkle parsley over finished dishes for a fresh touch.

Optimize vegetable intake. Blood Type A individuals thrive on a diet rich in vegetables. Incorporate a variety of fresh, organic vegetables into every meal. Leafy greens like spinach, kale, and Swiss chard are excellent choices. Add these greens to smoothies, salads, and sautéed dishes. Root vegetables like carrots and sweet potatoes can be roasted or added to soups and stews.

Focus on lean, digestible proteins. While plant-based proteins are preferred, small amounts of fish and poultry can also be included. Opt for easily digestible fish like salmon and mackerel, which are rich in omega-3 fatty acids. Prepare fish by grilling, baking, or steaming to retain nutrients. For poultry, choose organic, free-range chicken or turkey and cook using healthy methods like roasting or grilling.

Adjust baking recipes. When baking, substitute wheat flour with alternative flours like almond flour, coconut flour, or gluten-free blends. These flours are suitable for Blood Type A and can be used in cakes, cookies, and bread. Use flax eggs (ground flaxseed mixed with water) as a substitute for regular eggs in vegan baking. Sweeten desserts with natural sweeteners like maple syrup or agave nectar instead of refined sugar.

Create nutrient-dense smoothies. Smoothies are a convenient way to incorporate a variety of beneficial ingredients. Use a base of almond milk or coconut water, and add leafy greens, fruits, and plant-based proteins. Include ingredients like spinach, berries, chia seeds, and spirulina. Blend until smooth for a nutrient-packed breakfast or snack.

Experiment with new recipes. Adapting to a Blood Type A diet may require trying new recipes and ingredients. Explore different cuisines that naturally align with the dietary guidelines, such as Mediterranean or Asian dishes. These cuisines often emphasize plant-based ingredients, healthy oils, and a variety of vegetables.

By making these adjustments and substitutions, recipes can be adapted to fit the Blood Type A diet while maintaining flavor and nutritional value. This approach ensures that meals are both enjoyable and supportive of optimal health for Blood Type A individuals.

# Conclusion

Embracing the Blood Type A Food List involves a commitment to understanding and prioritizing the unique dietary needs associated with this blood type. By focusing on foods that are beneficial and avoiding those that can cause harm, individuals with Blood Type A can experience significant improvements in their overall health and well-being.

The Blood Type A diet emphasizes a plant-based approach, rich in vegetables, fruits, legumes, and whole grains. These foods provide essential vitamins, minerals, and antioxidants that support the immune system, enhance digestion, and promote a healthy metabolism. Incorporating beneficial proteins such as tofu, tempeh, and certain fish can further ensure that dietary needs are met without causing undue stress on the digestive system.

Avoiding harmful oils and fats is crucial for Blood Type A individuals. These can lead to inflammation, digestive issues, and other health complications. Opting for healthier alternatives like olive oil and flaxseed oil can provide the necessary fats without the associated risks.

Incorporating micronutrient essentials into the diet ensures that Blood Type A individuals receive the vitamins and minerals needed for optimal health. Foods rich in vitamin A, vitamin C, folate, iron, calcium, magnesium, zinc, and omega-3 fatty acids should be prioritized to support various bodily functions and prevent deficiencies.

By following the Blood Type A Food List, individuals can achieve a balanced and nutritious diet tailored to their specific needs. This personalized approach to eating not only helps in managing weight and energy levels but also contributes to long-term health benefits such as reduced inflammation, improved immune function, and enhanced mental clarity.

Implementing these dietary changes can lead to a more vibrant and energetic lifestyle. It is important to remember that consistency is key, and making gradual adjustments to incorporate the recommended foods will make the transition smoother and more sustainable. As individuals begin to experience the positive effects of the Blood Type A diet, they are likely to feel more motivated to continue on this path.

Ultimately, the Blood Type A Food List provides a comprehensive guide to eating in a way that aligns with the body's natural tendencies and promotes optimal health. By making informed choices and prioritizing beneficial foods, individuals with Blood Type A can enjoy a healthier, more fulfilling life.

www.ingramcontent.com/pod-product-compliance
Lightning Source LLC
Chambersburg PA
CBHW051605250726
48653CB00004BA/1338